Female Survivors of Sexual Abuse

Sexual abuse against females is a serious problem in society and there is a need for a greater understanding of the presentation and treatment of adult survivors of sexual abuse. In *Female Survivors of Sexual Abuse*, Christine Baker combines her clinical experience with an innovative approach to the treatment of this problem.

Female Survivors of Sexual Abuse addresses the experience of 180 female adults who were sexually abused in childhood, and provides detailed analyses and treatment approaches. The subject matter is presented in an accessible and compassionate way, imparting personal opinion and experience. It covers:

- female survivors: their stories, and the evidence
- integration, the alliance and the therapist
- the survivors' journey to recovery
- the families, disclosure and the role of the mother

This book enables the reader to "enter" the experience of the survivors and follow their progress to recovery, while highlighting the ever-changing state of knowledge in this difficult area. It will be invaluable to practitioners and students of clinical psychology, counselling, and psychiatry.

Christine D. Baker is a consultant clinical psychologist practising in Jersey, providing a specialist service for survivors of childhood sexual abuse. She is the co-editor of *Psychological Perspectives on Sexual Problems*, Routledge, 1993.

Female Survivors of Sexual Abuse

An integrated guide to treatment

Christine D. Baker

First published 2002 by Brunner-Routledge
27 Church Road, Hove, East Sussex BN3 2FA

Simultaneously published in the USA and Canada
by Taylor & Francis Inc.
29 West 35th Street, New York, NY 10001

Brunner-Routledge is an imprint of the Taylor & Francis Group

© 2002 Christine D. Baker

Typeset in Times by Mayhew Typesetting, Rhayader, Powys
Printed and bound in Great Britain by MPG Books Ltd, Bodmin

British Library Cataloguing in Publication Data
A catalogue record for this book is available from the British Library

Library of Congress Cataloging-in-Publication Data
Baker, Christine D.
    Female survivors of sexual abuse / Christine D. Baker.
        p.   cm.
    Includes bibliographical references and index.
    ISBN 0-415-13983-X – ISBN 0-415-13984-8 (pbk)
    1. Adult child sexual abuse victims. I. Title.

    RC569.5.A28 B35 2002
    616.85'8223906–dc21

                                                    2001052870

ISBN 0-415-13983-X (hbk)
ISBN 0-415-13984-8 (pbk)

To all the female survivors I have had the privilege to work with, for making this book possible.

Also to my husband David, for showing me that a loving and mutually respectful relationship is possible.

RESTLESS

Days propel spasms of tears
discharging all concealed fears
Restless in mind, want to hide
all too often thought I tried

Again I sit all on my own
no good for the body or bone
Restless in mind, tired brain
it's a wonder I am still sane

Scared to plunge and mingle
years drift by and still I tingle
Restless in mind, deep inside
emotions run high with the tide

My walls protect me for quiet
but are we ever ready to forget
Restless in mind, not to abide
in need of someone I can confide

Wish to be a bird and away fly
high up take clear air supply
Restless in mind, weep like rain
time to understand and explain

These final swoops shed the strings
off into the sky on great wings
Restless in mind, time to flee
Climb the horizon and to set free

A survivor

Contents

Illustrations

Acknowledgements

The first and foremost acknowledgement is to all the women survivors who have made this book possible. Without them and without the trust they placed in me to help them through their journey of recovery, this book would not have been written. Indeed, I am not only grateful to them for making it possible to put together a text that will hopefully inspire other professionals, but also for giving me the opportunity to develop and grow as a professional and human being.

I am equally indebted to my husband David. Without his staunch support, his unwavering belief in me and my project, and his patience at times of despondency—not to mention his endless resources in helping me with the administrative aspects of the book—I doubt that I would have completed my own journey. I would also like to thank my children, Leah and Alexis, for the respect and interest they have for my work and for the unconditional love they give me, which never fails to remind me of the important things in life. Indeed, I would like to thank all my family, and in particular, my father, for instilling in me the importance of hard work and belief in a personal vision.

Many other people I have been fortunate to know and work with have, in their own way, made this book possible. My boss, Ian Berry, has never failed to support me in my project and has been generous and patient when I have requested relevant professional training as well as time to complete the book. Without funding me to do the various courses abroad, which have given me the confidence to develop my training in schema-focused cognitive therapy, I would not have gained the necessary confidence to help my patients. A particular thank-you also goes to Sylvia Tillman, the librarian at the General Hospital where I work, who has been saintly in her patience and determination to conduct endless literature searches and acquire the reading that I needed. Thank you Sylvia.

It is to Padmal de Silva, my supervisor and mentor at the Institute of Psychiatry where I trained, that I owe my appreciation of the importance of sound theoretical models and the ability to produce clear and well-written formulations. He has been an excellent role model, both as a clinician and an academic. I would also like to thank Stephen Frosh who kindly agreed to talk to me when I was faced with a dilemma about how to present the book, and for whom I have the greatest respect for his own work in the field of child sexual abuse (CSA).

I would like to express my thanks and appreciation to the Jersey community for its support and positive feedback during the preparation of this book. In particular, I am very indebted to Ian Rogan who sacrificed his weekend to help me input my data and prepare the statistical information for the descriptive analysis in Chapter 4. Christine Herbert, a reporter for Jersey's newspaper, has the positive qualities that exemplify the professional and responsible aspects of media coverage. I would like to thank her for the very balanced and informative piece she contributed to the paper based on the interview we did on survivors of CSA and the book.

I would like to pay homage to Mo Henderson who is a lady of great wisdom and inspiration. Many of the women I have treated have attended her workshops on "mindfulness" which proved to be an invaluable adjunct to the work we did. Her in-depth knowledge in blending cognitive techniques with Zen Buddhist philosophy has been for me a great source of inspiration, courage, and patience at times of self-doubt.

I would also like to pay tribute to my close friends and colleagues, Jane Ussher, Eileen Engleman, and Cecily Hart. They have all followed my journey in the preparation of this book with genuine interest, and provided much needed support, both through their friendship and their experience in working with women. In particular, I owe a great deal to Jane Ussher, whose expertise in women's issues has given me the greatest insights into understanding their dilemmas, struggles, and strengths.

Last but not least, I would like to thank the editorial staff at Routledge who have been patient, supportive, and always helpful and available when I needed them.

Christine Baker
October 2001

Foreword

This is a powerful and moving book, which delves deeply into the experiences of women who have survived childhood sexual abuse to uncover the painful reality of their long-term negotiation of sexuality, identity, and mental health. Yet it also provides a hopeful vision of recovery through detailed accounts of sensitive therapeutic interventions and women's own resilience. This is important, groundbreaking work, which will have a significant impact on our understanding of the long-term effects of child sexual abuse, and on the ways in which we can ameliorate the pain and suffering of women survivors.

Reading this book from start to finish without a break, I was left with a feeling of profound sadness, but also of empowerment. The personal accounts of sexual abuse and family relationships that Christine Baker documents touch the soul in a way that bald statistics on CSA prevalence rates never can. But these statistics are also there and are a vital part of the case that is made: childhood sexual abuse is a pervasive problem in our society, affecting up to thirty percent of women. Reported cases are merely the tip of the iceberg—as is eloquently argued, the majority of survivors never disclose sexual abuse, either as children, or in adulthood. And if they do, we often don't want to hear. As parents, teachers, clinicians, family members, and friends we can so easily turn a blind eye. Our silence compounds the impact of the abuse. In this book, Christine Baker breaks the silence, she does not turn away, but rather documents women's experiences, and provides us with an insight into her own therapeutic work, where she is able to empathise, to hold each woman's pain, and through her skilled judgement and a range of clinical strategies, facilitate a journey of recovery. It is not an overstatement to say that it is inspirational.

This book will be indispensable to clinicians working with individuals who have been sexually abused as children, in both the coverage of the academic literature on the subject, and in the practical suggestions of how to ameliorate long-term problems. It will also be of interest to women survivors—the personal accounts provide an avenue for identification, and the stories of successful resolution of difficulties, a model of hope. If it

encourages survivors to seek therapeutic help in order to address the impact
of sexual abuse, and thus to move forwards positively, it will have served its
purpose.

However, whilst sexual abuse is the focus of this book, it is not only of
relevance to those whose life or work has been touched by such experiences.
The model of clinical intervention provided here, schema focussed cognitive
behavioural therapy, described through detailed case studies, and reflexive
analysis on the part of the author, will be of interest to clinicians working in
many areas of mental health. Christine Baker provides us with an exemplary model of the scientist-practitioner in action. Drawing on extensive
research and clinical literature, as well as her own training in cognitive
behavioural, psychodynamic and humanistic therapy, she has developed a
systematic approach to clinical intervention with women. However, this is a
scientist-practitioner with a heart; a clinician who states that "the relationship" is at the heart of her work with clients. This is not merely
rhetoric; it is illustrated through insightful case studies where the strength
and power of the therapeutic relationship shines out from the writing. And
this is presented as a two-way relationship—a clinician whose personal
growth has been profoundly affected by her experiences with her clients,
and who can acknowledge and learn from her mistakes, as well as take
pleasure and joy in her successes. This is a model for all trainee clinical
psychologists to follow—indeed, for all clinicians, no matter how long
qualified.

I would like to end this foreword on a personal note. I first met Christine
many years ago, when we were both working at a large teaching hospital in
London. Christine was a clinical psychologist specialising in psychosexual
issues, with a long waiting list and the almost unheard of reputation as
someone whose clients never failed to attend for sessions. I was a trainee
clinical psychologist, struggling to find a model I could believe in. At the
time I was grappling with the seemingly impossible contradiction of wanting to work clinically with women who experienced mental health problems, whilst theoretically adopting a critical feminist standpoint. I saw
women's difficulties as being largely located in social context, with the
pathologisation of problems on the part of psychology or psychiatry merely
adding to personal pain, rather than alleviating it. It was impossible to have
faith in what I was attempting to do   practice with conviction as a clinical
psychologist. In contrast, Christine had complete faith and belief in her
work. I tried to model myself on her for a time, attempting to do cognitive
behavioural work, but it didn't work for me. So after much deliberation, I
decided not to practice clinically any more, and confined myself, for many
years, to academic critique.

Reading this book, seeing the way in which sensitive schema-based
cognitive behavioural therapy does not pathologise women, and can indeed
incorporate a sophisticated critique of power relations, and an under-

standing of the importance of the dynamics of family life, my faith in clinical psychology is renewed. But I am also reminded of the importance of passion and conviction on the part of the therapist—we must believe in what we do, as Christine does, or our work will not be effective. For some time I have been contemplating further therapeutic training and a return to clinical work. This book has provided the final impetus—reading it becoming a literal moment of epiphany that I am very grateful for. I have every confidence that it will inspire others equally: clinicians to work with women who have been sexually abused; clinical psychologists to seek post-qualification training to further develop their skills; and women to seek help from sensitive clinicians.

The silence surrounding child sexual abuse has now been broken. It is time to do something about it—time we listened, and took seriously, the children who are being abused, but also the adult survivors, in order to help them to overcome their pain. Christine Baker has been able to do this in her work. It is now time for others to follow her lead, and to do the same.

Jane M Ussher, November 2001
Associate Professor, School of Psychology,
University of Western Sydney, Australia

Part I

Introduction: Survivors' stories and the evidence

Chapter 1

Background to the book and its aims

HISTORICAL CONTEXT

To say that the writing of this book has been the most challenging, and ultimately the most satisfying project of my professional life to date, would be an understatement. The best way I can describe it is in terms of an odyssey that has encompassed all of the joys, frustrations, and despondencies, along with the isolation, personal development, and exhilaration which can be experienced having embarked on a journey in uncertain but rich terrain. More than a decade ago, as a clinical psychologist working in a teaching hospital in west London and having recently completed my training, I had barely given the issue of childhood sexual abuse (CSA) much thought. In retrospect, it seems to me now as though it was a fact of life that people, both professional and lay, were aware of but for some reason had not yet entered their consciousness to a great degree.

Knowing what I know today, having treated hundreds of female survivors of CSA, and having researched the topic in great depth, I can only be amazed that even as recently as fifteen years ago, how low down on society's agenda was the silent suffering of people who as children had experienced the ultimate betrayal. My personal view is that at long last the issue of CSA is now firmly embedded in our consciousness but it is also my belief that it continues to be a complex topic that gives rise to a host of competing and emotive attitudes, which, in recent times, have heralded an unprecedented level of interest in the topic in many quarters of society. As professionals, we are currently undergoing a much awaited period of development in terms of our knowledge and understanding of the extent of CSA, and most importantly of the validation of survivors' experience. I believe that we owe a great deal to the pioneers, researchers, and clinicians of the early and mid-1980s—such as Finkelhor, Courtois, and Jehu—who put the topic of CSA on the map, so to speak, of academic enquiry and clinical awareness. As a result, over the past decade, survivors of CSA have finally been encouraged to have a voice and begin their journey of validation and recovery. Indeed, Finkelhor and Browne's (1985, 1986) proposed traumagenic model to explain the long-term effect of sexual abuse was a significant contribution in our initial attempts to conceptualise the impact of CSA and so begin to understand the nature of the suffering of survivors.

The historical context of the impetus and route that led to the writing of this book began with my interest in sexual dysfunction and the difficulties that led to sexual dissatisfaction. The initial interest in male sexuality (Baker and de Silva, 1988; Baker, 1993) inevitably encompassed female sexuality and its discontents (Baker, 1992). Indeed, as a basic grade clinical psychologist I realised that I was developing a keen interest in understanding female sexuality and I was fortunate to work in a hospital setting that allowed me to see women who were referred from a variety of medical, surgical, psychiatric, and therapeutic sources. Very soon, I became aware of the frequency with which many of the women who were complaining of sexual dissatisfaction were also reporting experiences of childhood sexual abuse. I was also made rudely aware that apart from the reassurance and support I could provide to these women, I was ill-equipped and lacking in the necessary knowledge with which to guide and inform them. I experienced both a profound sense of responsibility as well as a pressing professional and academic need to create a path that was to lead to the establishment, in Jersey, of a specialist service for survivors of sexual abuse, which ran concurrently with my own continual learning and development in the area of CSA.

AIMS

There are two central aims to this book, both of which are of equal importance and can best be subsumed under the rubric of "validating the experience of female survivors of CSA". Very frequent remarks that survivors make relate to their pain and anger at not having been believed when they disclosed their abuse as children, or when they were met with their families' ambivalence as adults. For those who did not have the resources or ability to disclose their abuse, their pain is about the lack of protection and detection either from their mothers, or society, and at times, both.

I have been asked whether there was a particular reason why I have omitted the experience of male survivors, and the simple answer is that the women who have presented for treatment have far exceeded in number their male counterparts. Indeed, the relatively few male survivors of CSA whom I have treated leads me to believe that this is an area that requires urgent attention, not least in understanding the reasons for which men may be reluctant to come forward, their individual ways of coping with the abuse, and the types of long-term effects they experience.

The first aim has been to impart to other professionals the wealth of knowledge I have gained as a clinician who has treated hundreds of female survivors of CSA in the past decade. I sincerely hope that this book will succeed in offering guidance and valuable insights to those in training or contemplating work with survivors of CSA, be they psychologists, social workers, counsellors, or those working in many of the vital voluntary or charitable organisations. For those who already have expertise in the treatment of CSA, or who have an academic interest in women's issues, the extended case studies in the book will hopefully provide additional insights or, indeed, motivate further practice, research, or critique.

The second aim has been to provoke further interest in the area of CSA, which, in my opinion, is still in its infancy. The many changes that have occurred in the past decade, in terms of our knowledge and the increased profile of the topic, confirm that we have still a long way to go before we can claim to understand fully what it means to have been sexually abused. For example, we have yet to subject the experience of those who have suffered minimal effects as a result of CSA to scientific enquiry, both in terms of prevalence and individual differences. Another area that requires attention, urgently, relates to paedophiles and child sex offenders. The existing work is in its early stages, as is the evaluation of the nature of perpetrators. As regards the latter, I refer to the relationship of the perpetrator to the survivor. Although there is general consensus that most CSA is perpetrated by men (see Chapter 15), and also that most perpetrators are likely to be a family member (see Chapters 2, 4, and 13), there continues to be conflicting information about their relationship to the survivors. In the UK, for example, figures published in a survey by the NSPCC (1990) suggested that 25 per cent of all CSA was committed by natural fathers. Interestingly, the NSPCC's figures from a similar survey in 2000 were reported in a rather sensational article in *The Independent on Sunday* (19 November 2000), in which brothers and stepbrothers were focused on as being the main culprits of CSA, accounting for almost 40 per cent of all attempted CSA. Consistent with the earlier findings, natural fathers were responsible for just over 20 per cent of all CSA. Clearly, there is a great deal more we need to learn about the relationship of perpetrators to the children they abuse, particularly because the picture is further complicated by the suggestion that in the clinical setting survivors frequently report abuse by fathers and step fathers (see Chapter 4).

STYLE

In order to succeed in fulfilling the above aims I considered that it would be important to create a "different" kind of book and I was aware that I was taking a risk in doing so. In other words, I wanted to ensure that the reader could access with ease and, hopefully, interest, the richness of the context within which survivors achieved their freedom from the experience of CSA.

In the event, this did not prove difficult because, from the moment of its conception, six years ago, the book naturally evolved from being a dry academic text to one, which, I would like to believe, imparts the human and powerful dynamics of the therapist–client relationship. Indeed, I can now assert that it would have gone against my integrity to present this book in any other way.

So what makes this book so different? First, it is written in the first person which is not a usual mode of writing in academic texts. The reason for this is to minimise the dichotomy between therapist and client and to maximise the human and interactive element that was in process during the writing of the book. Secondly, the book contains personal information about myself which relates to my own development and growth during the course of treating the women who came to me for help, and also during the preparation of the manuscript. There are a few reasons why I chose to include this. I wanted to express the humbling effect that working with very brave women had on me, and so it seemed to go against the grain to elevate myself to the position of a detached and all-knowing observer. I also wanted to share, in the best way I knew, the degree of respect and gratitude I have for these women, who not only allowed me the privilege of sharing their experience but who also contributed to my own growth.

A further distinguishing mark of this book is the manner in which I have treated the three case studies in Chapters 9, 10, and 11. These chapters are for me the core and heart of the book because it was my primary aim to validate the experience of the female survivors. I wished to distance myself from a reductionist model that presents a clinical case as an exhibit of "how it is done". What I have learned is that nothing in this life is simple and, therefore, it was important to create the best medium within which to allow the reader to appreciate the complexity of survivors' experience and their journey to recovery. With this in mind, I have integrated both a narrative as well as an analytic approach to the description, conceptualisation, formulation, and treatment issues of each case study. I have also made every effort to convey the interactive nature of the intervention approaches in the hope that my arguments on the therapist's characteristics in Chapter 7 would be clearly illustrated.

STRUCTURE OF THE BOOK AND HOW TO USE IT

The chapters in this book are presented in such a manner as to render it a versatile text that can be used in different ways. For the more advanced and experienced practitioner in the area of CSA, the book may be used as an informative text that can be referred to according to individual interest in any of the topics I have covered. It can also be a reference text for anyone involved in academic study or research.

For those who are just embarking on the study of CSA, the book follows a logical progression, beginning with the first of five parts. Part I comprises five chapters, and the aim here is to present a coherent background as an introduction to the parts that follow. Chapter 2 ("Fact and fiction") is divided into two sections, with the first providing an initial acquaintance to the three women—Victoria, Rose, and Florence whose journey to recovery is addressed later in the book. Their verbal report represents a powerful and emphatic start into the personal meaning of CSA, and I deliberately refrained from providing immediate formulations and conceptualisations. This was done in order to maximise the reader's appreciation of the chapters that follow and to prepare the ground for the in-depth focus of each individual case in Chapters 9, 10, and 11. The second part of Chapter 2, which deals with the media, was included in order to illustrate the part it has to play in terms of its potentially positive as well as negative effects on survivors of CSA.

Chapter 3 provides the historical background to the development of empirical work in the area of CSA and will highlight the relative recency of such work, as well as the difficulties encountered when attempting to define and measure the prevalence of CSA. Chapter 4 sets out the context of my own work and observations based on 180 female survivors of CSA. For ease of reference, I have included in the form of tables the breakdown of relevant variables related to both the demographic characteristics of the survivors as well as the abuse. The latter are summaries of the descriptive relevant statistics that may help the reader to gain an overall view of the general profile of a group of survivors who were referred for psychological treatment. The last chapter in Part I provides an in-depth discussion of the long-term effects of CSA. The information in this chapter aims to provide the reader with the understanding and insights that have been proposed so far, and will help to provide the necessary background for the formulations that follow in Part III of the book.

Part II paves the way for Part III, which is the central core of the book. Chapter 6 introduces the importance of model integration when treating survivors of CSA and discusses the reasons for this. In this chapter, I also make a case for the importance of the therapeutic relationship as being the one constant and dynamic factor in the development of a therapeutic alliance. I argue that the latter is the main vehicle towards positive change and I also explain why this is particularly vital when treating survivors of sexual abuse. Chapter 7 extends this discussion to examine the therapist's characteristics, and it is here that I reveal personal information about myself. Indeed, it is here that I pay my tribute to the clients whom I have had the privilege to treat, in terms of the development I have undergone, which has in turn affected my therapeutic practice.

I have already anticipated a possible criticism that Chapters 7 and to some extent 6 are idiosyncratic, given their personal nature. I would argue, however, as already mentioned earlier in this introduction, that this was the only way I could conceive of putting together a book that would be an honest and humble account, and also one that would be able to provide the important insights that I have gained during a decade's work with hundreds of women who have been sexually abused.

Part III comprises four chapters. Chapter 8 provides an introduction to the three-stage working model that I adopt when treating survivors. This is an extension of the previous two chapters and illustrates the model integration process. As I have already indicated, Chapters 9, 10, and 11 represent the main focus of the book, in which Victoria, Rose, and Florence are given extended attention. Here the reader can consolidate the information gained so far and can follow "in action", so to speak, each individual story from initial introduction to therapy, until final resolution of their abuse and eventual growth and independence. In the Appendix at the end of the book, the interested reader will find a list of relevant reading for the therapeutic techniques and conceptualisations that are discussed in the treatment of the three women.

I have dedicated Part IV to an examination of the families of origin of survivors of CSA. There is now growing consensus that the family of origin, and in particular mothers, have a crucial part to play both in the onset of CSA and the degree of long-term effects survivors are likely to experience. In Chapter 12 I accord particular attention to mothers and I would like to issue a warning from the outset that this may prove to be a sensitive area of discussion. However, I would also like to reassure the reader that I had no particular wish to downgrade mothers, my primary motivation being to express the experience of the women whom I have seen. Indeed, if anything, mothers have been portrayed as being powerful and very influential in either helping or hindering their daughters' recovery.

Finally, Part V concludes with two chapters that highlight the ever changing nature and degree of knowledge we are acquiring in the study of CSA. Books written on the treatment of sexual abuse in the 1980s or even the early 1990s will not have included the issue of false memory, or the treatment of child sex offenders. In Chapter 14 the reader will be able to follow a summary of the recovered/false memory debate, which became established by 1995. In Chapter 15 the closing remarks for the book attempt to address survivors' repeated questions about why people abuse children and what can be done about this. A case will be made for the fact that responsibility for the prevention of CSA lies primarily with society as a whole and, of course, the family.

Chapter 2

Fact and fiction

A TRILOGY: THE STORIES OF THREE WOMEN

Victoria

I have very mixed-up feelings about my childhood, but worst of all I feel very bad about myself. To the outside world I appear to be confident, together, and the person people feel they can come to and confide their problems. Inside, I often see an ugly, sad person who is unable to sustain relationships or ever feel properly loved. If people say they care for or love me, I think they have ulterior motives and I generally find it very difficult to trust anyone. I feel especially guilty when I look at what I have achieved and think that maybe I am making a fuss about nothing, because so much time has passed since I left my house, my family, and all other connections with the first eighteen years of my life.

I don't remember very much of the first five years of my life. I suppose my first memory is of my brother being brought to the house with my mother and father from the hospital where he was born. I remember thinking that it would be good to have someone to play with and not feel so lonely because my parents were often preoccupied with their own relationship (a very difficult one), or with their own socialising, work, and other aspects of their lives, to spend any time with me. I had a succession of nannies who for one reason or another never seemed to last very long and I remember the sadness I used to feel when they left, especially if I had built a bond with them. My hope of having a baby brother to look after and later play with was soon dashed, as he was a rather sickly baby, and my mother (who I now realise suffered with post-natal depression) became extremely anxious and would spend what seemed to be an eternity with him in her bedroom, while the family doctor seemed to be constantly paying visits. I was not allowed to intrude, let alone touch my brother, and I started to feel a great feeling of rejection and even more loneliness than ever before.

This situation must have gone on for at least the first three years of my brother's life and my only real solace during that time was to be found in my maternal grandfather, but only at first . . . He used to be a seldom visitor to our home before my brother was born but then he lost my grandmother, and this worsened my mother's depression. The good thing for me (or so I felt at the time) was that he came to live with us because he had a heart condition and my parents felt he would be better looked after with us. The first year after his arrival was probably the happiest I had experienced up to then. Nanny had now become my mother's right-hand help with my brother and so my grandfather would take me out for walks in the local park and even took me to the fair, an activity frowned on by my parents. He would also read me stories at bedtime, help me with my homework, and generally seemed interested in me; at last, I felt I had a friend. Because we lived in a remote part of town, it was rare for friends to come over after school, and in any case I was a rather quiet, introverted sort of child and did not make friends easily. Books and comics had been my loyal friends and some years later my mother commented that I appeared happier with my books than being with people; if she had only taken the trouble to get to know me she would have found out how lonely and rejected I felt and that I longed to be nurtured by her and also my father.

My parents must have been relieved that I was no longer asking for attention, and whatever guilt they may have had about neglecting me was clearly being appeased by knowing that I was "taken care of". This is exactly what my grandfather did; he took care of me in what I know now to be a very inappropriate and even damaging way. I still bear the scars of his actions, but most of all his betrayal. It was my seventh birthday when his behaviour towards me started to change and, at first, I did not understand what was going on. I remember him going to a lot of trouble with choosing my presents and he even arranged for a birthday cake to be delivered and had bought some balloons. I was so incredibly happy when we all sat down to a small birthday party meal and even my little brother was with us in his high chair. Then when it was bedtime, my grandfather came into my room to tuck me in as he had been doing for some months, only this time he didn't just kiss me on the cheek as he used to, but slid his hand under the covers and his hand was on my vagina and his fingers started to move around. I cannot really describe how I felt. It was a mixture of surprise, confusion, fear, and total incomprehension of what was happening: Grandfather was different and he was doing something that did not seem right. I wriggled around trying to free myself from his hand but he continued to stroke me all over my body and I felt his heavy breathing on my face. I was frozen. Then he started to whisper in my ear, saying: "You know you are my favourite and I want to show you how much I really love you; you are my special granddaughter and I want you to feel good. This will be our little secret and you must not tell anybody else, or they will be very jealous." After what seemed to be an eternity, he stopped and left the room. The feeling of loss, bewilderment, and unfamiliarity with what had just happened was to haunt me for many, many years. But the worst feeling that night was a sense of darkness that surrounded me and the sensation of sliding into a deep, lonely hole where nobody could reach me.

After that night, my grandfather, who I had got to love so very much, started doing more and more of these unfamiliar things and his kindly face became, for me, that of a monster. What had I done wrong? Was I so bad that I deserved him to do these things to me? He said I was special to him, so maybe I did something to make him give me this "special treatment". I tried to be really good and distract him (when his face would change) by bringing toys out to play with or by telling him excitedly about what I had done at school. But he was less interested than he had been, and when my parents were out for the evening (my mother was recovering from her depression), and he babysat, the nightmare would start all over again. Not only would he "touch" me when I was in bed but now he started to unzip his trousers and took his penis out. The first time he did this I was sitting on his lap. I could feel him doing something to himself and then he took my hand and placed it on this squeegee, soft thing which then started to change and become harder. His grip on my hand was firm and he made me rub his penis until something liquid covered my hand. Again, he whispered in my ear that he loved me and that I was his very special little girl and that I had been very good. I hated being good! He also said that time: "You know this is our secret, but even if you ever told anyone, they will not believe you and they will hate you for it."

This is what became of the next two of the formative years in my early development. If I was lonely before my grandfather joined our family, now I was lonely and very frightened, ashamed, and felt so different from other children. Losing my grandfather who I came to love, to this new "monster", was so unutterably bleak that I developed ways of "cutting myself off from the experience", by imagining I was somewhere else, far more sunnier and safer, where he could not reach me. I think I must have learned by heart every intricate pattern on the carpet and the curtains, not to mention how many there were.

So what of my mother? Why was she not there to observe and protect? This question still wounds me, especially as she and my father were only too happy to let my grandfather take over. Looking back, they were not bad people, only very unhappy with each other and very preoccupied with their work, with my brother's health, and with life's difficulties. Now I realise that my greatest loss was not being close to my mother, who while she made sure I had the right clothing, education, and nourishment, failed to nourish my spirit. I still hunger for true love and nurturing, and if it comes my way I have no appropriate mechanism to recognise it. My impoverished self-esteem can only attract those who seek to crush it further.

My ordeal at the hands of my grandfather ended when he died of a heart attack when I was nearly nine years old. Although at the time I felt a sense of relief, this was to give way to long-term feelings of guilt, shame, and responsibility for what had happened to me. I felt particularly guilty that I never had the courage to tell my parents, although I realise now that in retrospect it is easy to recriminate oneself.

After his death I threw myself into my school work, and although things in our household started to improve and I could now start to develop a relationship with my brother, I had an inner burning ambition to leave home as soon as possible, education being my passport to freedom from the past; or so I thought.

I am now a successful professional and I am independent financially. I live in a different part of the country to my parents but I see them about two or three times a year, when I go to visit. My mother continues to be a frail woman as regards her moods and her anxiety, and my father is still as unapproachable as he was, but perhaps slightly more interested in my life than he used to be. I still say very little about myself, and to this day they have no idea about what grandfather did, and I don't think I will ever tell them. So, to the outside world, I am a successful, working, single woman, who is level-headed, and independent, if somewhat of a loner. Although I feel comfortable with listening to others and even imparting some advice, I am loath to disclose anything of any consequence about myself, in case my persona becomes undermined and I then "lose" my grip on my security. The result is that I continue to be a lonely individual and, although I have had relationships with men, they usually end on a disastrous note and love continues to elude me.

Rose

We were what you would call a normal, average type of family. My parents were very religious and church on Sundays was an important ritual, which we all had to adhere to even if we, the children, protested or preferred to do other things instead. I was the middle child of three, the eldest being a boy and the youngest another girl. My parents were what you would call quite strict, but it was my mother we all feared the most. She would never hit us, but she could have a fierce temper and we knew, when she looked at us in that special angry tone of hers, not to talk back or disobey her. If we tried, she would not think twice to deprive us of something that was special to us, and she would stick to that no matter what. My father was quieter, and I think he was probably in fear of her as well because if he tried to contradict her she would dish out her verbal abuse to him as well. I often wondered how my mother could have this hold over him because she was not particularly well educated but he was a graduate, and from what I could gather, quite successful in his job as manager of a local firm.

My parents didn't seem to have much of a social life and religion played an important part in our lives, mainly instigated by my mother who was a devout Catholic. As you can imagine, sex was a taboo subject and I often wondered how we were conceived. Apart from the fact that my parents slept in separate beds, my mother would, given any opportunity, make remarks like: "Look at young women these days, they have no shame exposing their bodies like that to all and sundry; and as for her next door, I can't keep up with the number of men that seem to come in and out of her house—slut!" We were too young to understand what she meant at first, but later we knew better than to giggle about anything remotely sexual, let alone ask her any questions related to sex or intimate parts of the human body.

You can see that I am really avoiding coming to the point and saying exactly what it is I have come to seek help for. I find sex so disgusting and can't even bear to see my own body naked! I feel so guilty that I am depriving my husband of sex because he is such an understanding, loving, wonderful man. You see, my mother may have been twisted about sex, but it is my father who made sure that I too would become twisted about my own sexuality. I am not sure who is to blame, my mother for rejecting my father in the bedroom and for making us feel so ashamed about our sexual curiosity; my father, who took it upon himself to "teach me" (his words) the facts of life so that I would be in "safe hands first time around and ready for life"; or myself for being as weak as he was and not protesting enough, hitting out, or fighting to stop the nightmare from happening? The feelings of hatred and disgust inside me are sometimes too much to bear. Now I have to control these feelings because I have my own little girl and my biggest ambition is for her to grow into a healthy individual who loves herself and her body and who has a normal view of men and sex. She could never possibly see me resort to the sort of things I used to do to myself when I could not express how terrible, mixed up, and terrified I felt when "he" used to "teach me" the facts of life.

It all started one Sunday when we were all normally due to go to Mass. I was probably around nine years old at the time and I remember having been ill with a high temperature, and even my mother said I could be excused on this occasion from going to church. Unfortunately, for me, it seems that my father was also excused from going, saying that he would stay behind to be with me because he knew how much it mattered for my mother not to miss Mass. What happened that day has made me hate Sundays to this day; a day I usually busy myself in the house, furiously cleaning and tidying and avoiding any pleasurable activity. I am still avoiding coming to the point aren't I? I have never before been able to admit to myself what happened, let alone discuss it with a total stranger. In fact, I am so angry that having kept this horror under lock and key for all these years (thirty two of them!), now there is little I can do about the images that come to haunt me. I can certainly not resort to harming myself like I used to, with razors or pins. You probably think I am mad, but scratching my arms and legs was the only way I knew of making things go quiet in my head and in my heart when "things" used to happen. Now I could never let my little girl see me do harm to myself; I want her to have the healthy role model I never had. You see, my father had intercourse with me. That Sunday when I was ill and he stayed with me, he came to my bed and brought me a drink of hot chocolate, which was my favourite. Then, I could not understand why, but he took his trousers off and slipped into the bed beside me. He cuddled me and said he would keep me warm, and then he started to kiss me in a way I didn't like. I was starting to feel scared but this was nothing compared to what happened next. He hands were touching me all over my body and then he said that it was a father's duty to teach his little girl what happens when she grows older and meets men. He said these young men can be filthy, clumsy boys and they don't know what to do, but that he would show me the right way. There was nothing wrong in what he was going to do, but it was better that I say nothing to mother, who would not understand and would also not believe me. If I said anything to my brother or sister, they would hate me, so it was best to keep it our special secret. With that, his body was on top of me as I lay frozen, my mind a blank, and my eyes just staring at the ceiling. He parted my legs with his hands and then I felt myself being ripped open with the most excruciating pain I had ever felt. It seemed as though a sharp knife had stabbed me down below. Eventually, after what seemed for ever, he rolled over put his face on the pillow and started crying. I don't know how to really describe what I felt, except that I was in pain and then a warm liquid was trickling down my legs. I got up to go to the bathroom, I thought I had wet myself, and father said in muffled tones with his head still on the pillow, to go and wash myself off because mother would worry. I looked down and was terrified to see there was blood running down my legs. I went to the bathroom and locked myself in until my mother and siblings returned. I later heard my father tell my mother that I had been sick and he had to wash my sheets and that I was still poorly.

When I heard my father cry, I thought he regretted hurting me and that he would never think to "teach" me again. But this was not so. This unspeakable experience happened a few more times and could have happened even more if he had the opportunity to be left with me alone more often. When I look back, I see that he was clearly not remorseful at all. It is so difficult to try and explain all the emotions and thoughts that go through your head because, after all, I am no longer a child and I am sure I see things as I think I remember them now. All I can say is that if ever I had an inkling of anything like this happening to my daughter, I would be capable of murder. In fact I think I am overprotective of her.

Anyway, I suppose the greatest shock I had, even more than the pain my father inflicted on me, was when I had my first period at the age of just ten. Because the facts of life were of course never discussed (only savagely illustrated by my so-called father), when I discovered blood in my underwear I panicked because I thought my father may have damaged me more than I realised, or that I may be ill with something terrible. Although sworn to secrecy, my fear took over and I rushed to tell my mother I was bleeding. I half expected her (maybe wished her) to realise what my father had been doing, but instead she shook her head, handed me a towelling sanitary towel, and said that I was now a woman and could get pregnant: I knew, of course, what pregnant meant! It was no use asking my mother to reassure me or to properly explain what was going on, as she was hardly looking at me. Did this mean that when my father did what he did I could now have a baby in my tummy?

A couple of years later while looking through a magazine, the word incest appeared on the pages about a girl who was raped by her brother. It was then I properly realised how wrong it was what my father did to me, who for some reason I used to feel sorry about despite the things he put me through. Fortunately, when he realised about my periods, he put a stop to things, although he still continued to touch me where he shouldn't until I was fifteen. After all that happened to me, why I continued to stay at home until my early twenties I will never know. Another question that keeps coming into my head is, why did I never tell anyone? When I realised what incest was I would have had good reason to tell this horrible "secret" to someone—but who? My father's words would keep ringing in my ears, about not being believed, and being hated, and the thought of this was too terrible to contemplate. And so I stayed with my secret, until now that is.

Eventually, I found the courage to apply for a nanny's job abroad as I loved children and had taken a nursery course. The thought of a sexual relationship with anyone disgusted me totally but I longed to have children of my own and so, when I met my husband who is gentle and kind, I decided to overcome my feelings because the need to have a baby was much stronger. I explained my feelings about sex to him, and although I said I had some bad experiences in childhood, I did not then tell him exactly what happened. We did have sex, but it took several months before I could relax with him, usually after having some alcohol. I did not enjoy any of it, and then when I became pregnant I felt it was all worthwhile. Now I have my beautiful daughter I dread any form of close intimacy and have even suggested that we have separate beds, although I know how wrong this would be for him and for my daughter. What example would we give her? I know the time has come to face my past with honesty, although I hate the whole idea of it. If nothing else, I have to do it for my family.

Florence

I often feel grateful that, despite all I have suffered in my life, I can still hold on to happy memories of my very early childhood. It seems like a consolation for all the bad things that followed from when I was about ten years old. I have images of myself, my parents, and siblings (there are three of us altogether) when we used to be a really close family who did things together. We didn't have a lot of money but my father was a very hard-working carpenter and always used to say that being all together and taking care of one another was the most important thing. I really loved my father and although he always seemed so busy, he always managed to spend some time with us, and say encouraging things to make us feel loved and wanted. My mother was also a very hard-working woman and, when my youngest sibling reached the age of five, she decided to start working as an auxiliary nurse to help make ends meet. She was less affectionate and warm than my father, but she was conscientious and we always had a meal on the table and clean clothes for school.

My world seemed to fall apart when my father developed cancer and, after what seemed to be a very quick and brutal illness, he died when I was only nine years old. The whole family was shattered and even my mother, who always appeared so strong, seemed unable to cope. As the eldest daughter, I tried to be as helpful to my mother as I could, often missing school to do some cleaning and shopping and helping with my younger sister and brother. My mother now needed the money she could earn more than ever, and started to do night shifts at the hospital where she worked because this paid more money. I really missed her but I felt a sense of pride at being able to help her and babysit my younger siblings and help them get off to bed. I used to get very tired by the end of the evening and often missed doing my homework, which used to get me into trouble, but no one seemed interested in the struggle we were having at home. My mother was a proud woman, and I am sure she could have got some financial help from the government, but she would not hear of it when one of my aunts suggested it to her.

I was so happy when, about a year after my father died, my mother seemed to become more cheerful and more like her usual, coping self. Later she told us, rather shyly, that she had met a male nurse on her shifts who was divorced and who was a really nice person and wanted to meet us. I still missed my father such a lot and was not keen on meeting this person, but felt that if my mother was happy, then it could do no harm just to meet him. I remember clearly, to this day, the first time I met him. He was a rather large man with what seemed to be a jolly face, although I did not like the way he was so very quickly friendly and asking personal questions of us—I mean, we hardly knew him. He brought all our favourite sweets (my mother must have told him) and said he was very happy to have met our mother and hoped that in time we could get to like him. By the end of that first visit I knew I disliked him, but I was also very scared because my mother was clearly trying to get us to like him and I wondered if she would ever bring him to live with us. The thought filled me with horror and dread, but I could not tell you exactly why.

To cut a long story short, within a few months he married my mother and, of course, came to live with us and this was soon to change my life forever. His "jolly" face soon gave way to a face that was to inspire fear and even terror whenever he was in the room. He was a heavy alcohol drinker and, although at first this did not appear to affect our lives, within a few months he was taking more and more time off work and his temper knew no bounds. He would shout at all of us at the slightest thing and would throw things across the room; by the end of the first year with us, he was hitting my mother quite badly. But that is not all; the worst was to come, for me at least. One night, when my mother went out to work, he was sitting as usual on his favourite chair, and had been drinking for most of the afternoon. As usual, I had fed and helped my sister and brother to bed and was about to have a bath, when he pushed the bathroom door open and said it was about time he showed me how a real woman behaves. Everything happened so quickly, and I don't understand to this day why I was unable to escape and put a stop to the horrible things he did to me. He dropped his trousers and started playing with his penis, all the while walking towards me and cornering me against the wall. Then he grabbed my hair and pushed my head towards his "thing" and forced it into my mouth. It felt as though this assault was going on forever, and when he eventually ejaculated he left the room, making disgusting and obscene remarks as he was zipping up his trousers.

What can I say about how I felt, kneeling there on the bathroom floor, clutching at my dressing gown and furiously trying to wipe the smelly, sticky "gunge" from my face, feeling as though I wished I could disappear? I was nearly eleven and knew something about the facts of life from school and from gossiping with my friends, but I also knew that this was terribly wrong and should not have happened—it was wrong! I felt dirty, I felt stunned, and also very desperate about what to do next. My mother was already suffering, and telling her what happened would totally destroy her. At that time I could hardly recognise her. The strong, proud mother who seemed to flourish when my father was around was now a frightened woman, walking on eggshells, and in fear of the next blow, not to mention the insults and threats.

My stepfather's violation of me did not stop there. At every opportunity he would force me to give him oral sex and would say this was for my own good as I would be way ahead of other women when I started to have boyfriends. He had no respect for my privacy, and would constantly speak to me with sexual innuendoes, and made remarks about my developing body. He once tried to penetrate me but I said that I had started my periods and he would not want to make me pregnant. I was grateful and relieved that his drunken state seemed to accept this and that he remained content with using me to relieve his sexual urges in other ways. He said that if I ever told my mother, or anyone else, social services would put us all in a home and my mother would be destroyed. There was no way that I could have allowed this to happen. But his worst threat to me was that if I continued to "please" him he would then leave my younger sister, who was then eight, alone. This sent a shiver down my spine as I felt it my duty to protect my sister from such a horrible experience, and with this he made sure that I would allow myself to be used for his sexual gratification whenever he wished.

My ordeal continued for about three years, but as I was growing I became a rebellious teenager and would stay out late with my friends. These were the wilder bunch at school, and one in particular I felt very close to as she also indicated, although not in so many words, that her father was not all he should *be. Together we would smoke secretly and share wild dreams about how we would one day leave and never return. My stepfather (not worthy of his title) was deteriorating with his drinking and, although he tried to control me, I was becoming too unruly and aggressive to be controlled, and instead he took it out on my mother, telling her she was useless and that it was her fault I had become a slut. For this I felt very guilty because she did not deserve this abuse, but then I felt I had gone too far down the road of rebellion to turn back.*

Eventually, one day the bastard went too far in his beatings and my mother was admitted to hospital with a broken jaw and concussion from being repeatedly hit on the head. This seemed to bring me back to my senses and while in hospital I begged her to get out, saying that we would manage if she asked for help. I had heard from my close friend that her mother eventually went to a women's refuge, and although things were still pretty bad, she was beginning to build her life again. I said all this to my mother and she found the courage to press charges and place an injunction on him. He didn't accept this easily and continued his threats for a while, but my mother seemed to regain her lost dignity and courage and we moved to the refuge. I don't know what happened to the bastard, but one day the threats stopped and we never saw him again.

I can't say that my life became much happier straight away as a result. In fact, once my mother picked up enough of her strength I started accusing her and blaming her for what she allowed us all to go through. I felt I was becoming the abuser and felt very bad in myself about that, but it had all bottled up inside me for many years and I needed to punish her. One day I also threw at her the fact that her so-called husband had tried to rape me and that he would use me for his perverted acts. I will never forget the look of pain in her face when I said this and all she could say was how sorry she was and that she would try to make things up to me.

I didn't give her that chance: when my friend suggested we leave our town to start a new life elsewhere I jumped at the chance. With all that happened my education suffered badly, but at least I was now free to think only of myself and I knew I still had my good humour to see me along and the images of happier times in my early childhood. I can't say that my life was a bed of roses after I left home. I continued with my wild living and had a period of promiscuity and drinking too much, which left me feeling very bad about myself. Occasionally, I would be haunted by images of what the bastard did to me and I tormented myself over and over with self-recriminations about what I could have done to stop him abusing me. I have feelings of great sadness about how my life has turned out and what a disappointment I am to myself, but most of all to the memory to my dear dead father. I feel I am capable and smart and I could have achieved so much, but somehow I seem to be on self-destruction mode, when what I really long for is to have a close, happy family unit, and maybe recapture the brief happiness I once knew.

Deferring analysis

There is no doubt that these personal accounts convey a host of powerful and intense emotional and psychological experiences related to having suffered sexual abuse in childhood, and each memoir merits thorough and detailed analysis. After careful consideration, however, I decided that I would refrain from such analyses at this stage because I wished to present an emphatic opening to the book in order to maintain the momentum of the accounts until the "core" of the book is reached in Part III. I wish to reassure the reader that it has not been my intention to shock but rather to present experiences that were related to me during the course of therapy, and I have chosen them in order to illustrate the varying "face" of sexual abuse, while bearing in mind that it is, by no means, a total representation of what survivors experience.[1]

The impact of sexual abuse, in my experience as a therapist, can cover a whole range of behavioural, emotional, and psychological difficulties, which at one end of the spectrum can be termed "benign", and at the other end can be extremely severe (in Chapter 5 I examine closely the long-term effects). Although the choice of the personal accounts presented here was arbitrary and subjective, I believe that it is, nevertheless, a good representation of how the women conceptualise their experience and the effects it has had on them. My intention in presenting the accounts is that they would set the scene of the experience of sexual abuse and, in the first instance, be appreciated in their own right.

A further reason for deferring the analyses of the accounts is because their profound complexity requires a multifaceted and integrated approach to formulating and conceptualising the issues that survivors have raised. Consequently, these will be better appreciated and understood when they are tackled in depth, simultaneously with treatment interventions, following my discussions on model integration and therapist's characteristics (Chapters 6 and 7), which are central to the theoretical, but most importantly, clinical appreciation of each separate account.

Finally, the purpose of presenting the stories here is to highlight the apparent imbalance between what the survivors actually say and how the media represents them, and the misconceptions that continue to abound, not least the continued lack of appreciation (or denial) that most child sex offenders come from the survivors' background of family and friends. The following section examines some of the issues that relate to the role played by the media when tackling the topic of sexual abuse.

THE MEDIA

The growing media attention, in all its forms, in the topic of child sexual abuse (CSA) over the past fifteen years more than equals that accorded to it by academics. More importantly, the media appear to have adopted the subject to such a degree that, arguably, it currently constitutes one of the major areas of discussion, interest, concern and even anger or apparent revulsion, depending on which side of the fence one is sitting. In this part of the chapter I attempt to provide a brief discussion of the media's role in the documentation and reporting of child maltreatment in general, and CSA in particular. I also present my own reservations about the quality of such reportage in terms of its possible effects on adult survivors who are exposed to it.

Media reporting of CSA

A very informative critique on the media by Levey (1999) clarifies succinctly the limitations as well as potential uses of media reporting on child abuse in the USA. With respect to newspapers, he reflects that while fifty years ago stories on maltreated children would not be covered due to the "distasteful" nature of the topic, twenty-five years ago such stories were actively sought by the very same newspapers. Sadly, however, it was the scandal and shock element that aroused interest then, and similarly today, while newspapers cover some aspects of a story quite well, according to Levey they "nibble around the edges" of child maltreatment stories. Moreover, newspaper reporting can be bound up with financial, space, and vision constraints, which ultimately diminish the educational value of a piece. Because newspapers are daily sources of information, however, according to Levey (1999) advocates of crucial causes such as the reduction of CSA must not be deterred from approaching editors, as opposed to reporters, in applying pressure. For example, as a reporter himself, he advises that most editors would respond to being educated about the value of adopting, in some cases, a longer-term approach to a story, as opposed to the selling tactic of the one-off shock publication. Levey argues that if the drip-drip approach of providing informed articles that can have long-term beneficial effects on the consciousness of readers can be effectively "sold" to an editor, then the potential for more balanced reporting of child abuse is much increased.

Unfortunately, there is little evidence that rounded and balanced newspaper articles that inform and educate rather than shock are currently the norm in the UK. There are of course a few exceptions. One such example, in my opinion, was an *Independent on Sunday* article (19 November 2000), which reported the results of a survey by the NSPCC. Although I took issue with two aspects of this article (which I shall address shortly), the reporter took the trouble to provide an informative context within which to place the story. The article in question chronicled the false starts in the reporting of child maltreatment and CSA, as well as society's changing attitudes over the past forty years, starting up to the 1960s with public disbelief that cruelty and exploitation of children actually existed—namely the much publicised "battered child syndrome". Almost two decades later, the reporter argues, the public was still aghast at suggestions that men were capable of sexually abusing children barely able to walk. Indeed, the deaths of Maria Colwell in 1973 and of Jasmine Beckford a decade later highlighted the inadequacies of the social services system in protecting vulnerable children. Finally, the article discussed the current state of affairs, much influenced by changing attitudes towards the end of the 1980s, when the fact of sexual exploitation of children began to be accepted, particularly as a result of the backlash caused by the Cleveland and Orkney scandals, amongst others.

Unfortunately, however, the article fell into the very trap it was attempting to avoid. For a start, it utilised a sensationalist front-page title that purported to "reveal the truth about CSA in Britain's families". Clearly, not only are we a long way from feeling confident that we have the truth but, secondly, the reported assertion that it was siblings who were responsible for most intrafamilial sexual abuse, rather than fathers and stepfathers, was, in my opinion, quite misleading. While not wishing to underestimate the value of the survey, given that it was based on the disclosures of 2,869 young adults, the fact remains that disclosing abuse at the hands of a parent is a very grave issue for survivors. Certainly, as will become evident in the following chapters, the academic and clinical picture has generally pointed to fathers and stepfathers as accounting for a significant proportion of the perpetrators of CSA. Indeed, a recent publication by ChildLine (2000) reported that of the 115,000 children counselled by them between 1997 and 1998, about 20 per cent reported CSA. Although this report did not reveal the type of perpetrator, it did reassert that most abuse occurred in the home. Based on the sensationalist aspect of *The Independent on Sunday* report that most abuse occurs at the hands of siblings, would it not therefore be foolhardy to deduce that the 23,000 children of ChildLine's sample were abused by siblings alone?

One particularly good example of some newspapers' lack of balance and rounded information in articles on CSA—and their potential for not only misleading but also for causing severe distress to survivors and damage to clinicians' credibility—appeared in a tabloid paper in 1997. The article in question was clearly cashing in on the sensationalist reporting that "today's so-called counsellors can almost destroy a family". The story focused on the retraction of a patient's disclosure that her father had sexually abused her, this disclosure having been prompted by the alleged unethical practices of psychiatrists. While this story may have been true, no effort was made in the article to balance the information by distinguishing between different types of professionals who treat CSA, and the paper was clearly unable to differentiate between psychiatrists and counsellors. Indeed, the whole article was biased, ill-informed, and made no effort to reassure the public that not all therapists are unscrupulous. Most importantly, it did not make clear that, while the story reported an unfortunate event, most CSA does occur in the home, and that survivors should not be deterred from seeking treatment.

The discussion so far alerts us to the crucial responsibility the media has in informing the public about serious social issues and the fact that this responsibility does not appear to be always accorded due thought and concern. Indeed, Elvik (1994) asserts that "modern societies rely on the mass media for current and accurate information", and that "many people believe that if they hear news on television or radio, or read a particular account in a paper, that the material is factual and unbiased" (Elvik, 1994, pp. 133–134). If this is the case, then the issues I have just discussed and which, I believe, are shared by other caring professionals, should encourage us to remain vigilant by closely monitoring the changes in public attitudes as a result of media hype, which has the potential of distressing survivors and, of course, shaping public opinion. Moreover, it has the potential to cause rifts among the very professionals who are attempting to care for survivors.

Edwards and Lohman (1994) argued that those involved in the manage-ment of people who have been sexually abused are themselves affected by the media. Examining, for example, the impact of media narrative of incidents such as Cleveland, they point out that the media can appear to condemn the very people who diagnose CSA, causing divisions to the point that many frustrated professionals leave their chosen area of work. More recently, this state of affairs was clearly exemplified by the Waterhouse scandal, which revealed the alienation of those professionals who attempted to alert the relevant authorities about the incidents of sexual abuse in Welsh residential homes.

Finally, there is a further issue relating to the media's change of focus with respect to CSA that is worthy of note. Recently there has been a flurry in the reporting of paedophile activity involving the internet (e.g. *The Independent*, 14 February 2001). While such reporting is crucial in alerting us to the exploitation and possible abuse of children, there is a concern that a shift of focus may occur, whereby attention to the plight of survivors may give way to yet another change in the arena of media reporting and public interest. I do not for a moment suggest that such reporting should not take place, but that the mounting complexities involved in CSA, the nature of perpetrators, and the avenues for exploitation and offending should be addressed using comprehensive, well-informed, and rounded information.

Survivors' concerns and my experience

What is apparent to me, as a clinical practitioner involved in helping the women who have survived sexual abuse in childhood, is that despite the timely exposure of this endemic problem, there continues to exist a lack of adequate understanding and appreciation of what sexual abuse represents to those who have suffered it. Equally worrying is the fact that this misinformation can have disturbing effects on those survivors who come across it and experience either unwarranted or renewed anxiety.

Media hype can often be a disservice to those it is claiming to inform, and quite frequently this unprofessional and uneducated enthusiasm only succeeds in perpetuating or initiating undue distress that is very often seen in the consulting room. It must be pointed out, however, that this apparent ignorance highlights the degree to which a deeply ingrained societal aberration (which appears to observe no ethnic, cultural, religious, or historical boundaries) has managed to remain hidden until very recently. It is possible, therefore, that the flurry of current interest in the topic is society's opportunity to overcome a degree of guilt as a result of the absence of previous responsibility towards those who have no voice or those who, having dared to utter their distress, were either ignored or advised "to tell no one" lest it caused untold misery to the extended family.

As far as the general public is concerned (excluding those who have experienced CSA), information is mainly derived from hearsay, fantasy, and most frequently from these very same media-based representations, thus creating further confusion in the understanding of sexual abuse, not to mention feelings of "horror" and expressions of disbelief. Yet it is not unusual to hear that disclosure of sexual abuse by both children and adults may be a direct result of increased public awareness and media interest, and therefore it can help to bring forward those who need to be heard or to be helped. Although to an extent I share this view, as I attempted to explain in the previous section I also hold certain reservations about the type of material that is either published or broadcast. However my main concerns relate to the verbal reports of the women whom I have seen, who expressed both the positive and the negative aspects of media reporting.

With respect to the positive aspects of media publicity, I am referring to some rare but good dramatisations of the experience of sexual abuse, which have managed to tap into the survivors' perspective within a "normal context". By normal I do not mean ideal, but that the abuse was not perpetrated by a figure unknown to the abused—for example, an isolated attack in an otherwise ordered and loving environment, or in extreme circumstances that resulted in tragedy. When good drama represents the 'norm' in the portrayal of sexual abuse, it can facilitate identification with the character who was abused. Moreover, from the disclosure of some of the women I have seen, such drama or similar media representation can activate unresolved or unprocessed material linked to past abuse, which may promote the seeking of professional help. One needs to bear in mind, however, that there may be many others who are too anxious or reluctant to seek help, or who do not know where to seek it. In addition, even though most drama (if it is televised) is usually followed by "helpline" numbers, many may not make use of them, and if they do, it is uncertain what type of help they are offered, or if the venues suggested for help are accessible to those who do avail themselves of such a service.

The negative aspects of media publicity and representation in all its forms centre on the fact that, at best, they tend to offer arbitrary definitions and/ or guidance about how to identify abuse and its consequences, while at worst they tend to focus on the more extreme cases that in my view (based on work in this book) are not representative. The result is that the majority of those who have experienced sexual abuse feel alienated from such publications because they are unable to relate to them, or they may experience unwarranted distress, or indeed guilt, because their experience is not deemed to be worthy of concern. Equally, in some vulnerable individuals, material that is published without due caution, and that is based on dubious research methods, may cause unnecessary alarm. With respect to some of these points, let me give some specific examples, based on my experience.

The first example concerns a young woman who asked to be referred for psychological help because she read a magazine article discussing sexual problems, and it suggested that if a woman is experiencing lack of desire, one of the reasons may be that she was sexually abused as a child. This article was in one of the popular women's magazines, offering a brief "do-it-yourself" analysis of common sexual difficulties without the back-up of empirical information or balanced discussion. Clearly, not all such articles are irresponsible and misleading, but they do exist. The woman who was referred to me was an otherwise balanced individual who had been experiencing loss of libido for several months, having previously enjoyed her sexual relationship with her boyfriend. Reading the article with its reference to sexual abuse triggered a memory of when she was about twelve years old and an elderly neighbour made a few passing sexual comments to her and then once attempted to touch her breasts. She had no recollection of this incident intruding in her thinking. A combination of her unhappiness about her loss of sexual desire, the strain of her relationship, and then reading the article, triggered considerable distress. This was further exacerbated when light-heartedly mentioning the "neighbour episode" to a friend, the latter suggested that she should seek professional help.

This is one example of how popular media can contribute to unnecessary distress, because my formulation after having seen her was that the problem she was having was a result of communication difficulties in the relationship with her boyfriend and, later, his admission that he had had a brief affair. The "abuse" incident, once discussed in the sessions, did not appear to be a contributing factor and I was satisfied that it had been appropriately processed.

A second example concerns the observation that extreme publications and/or representations may alienate those who are unable to relate to them.

I am referring here to the storyline in a popular television soap some years ago, which focused on the sexual abuse of two sisters by their biological father. This was a powerful dramatisation that had some realistic aspects, such as the portrayal of the manner in which the father psychologically coerced his daughters into a sexually abusive situation. On the other hand, however, it also portrayed certain aspects that occur less frequently, such as the story's culmination in the murder of the perpetrator by one of his daughters. An additional factor was that domestic violence featured heavily in the script and several of my patients commented along the lines that "at least the women in this soap had no possibility of disclosing their abuse due to the constant threat of serious violence at the hands of their father and, therefore, they could absolve themselves from the responsibility of being subjected to abuse". In the majority of my patients' accounts, physical violence was not used by the perpetrator and the question that frequently haunts them is "why was I unable to stop it—after all, I never feared for my physical safety?" As professionals we know the answer to this question, which becomes a significant part of the therapeutic process because a constant rumination of survivors is the great burden of responsibility they bestow on themselves for being sexually abused.

A third observation I would like to make relates to the numerous documentaries in recent years that have concentrated on the uncovering of sexual abuse in residential institutions, and also news items and features concerning dangerous paedophiles and their activities. Although these frank publications may be argued to be timely and that they promote a sense of greater awareness on the part of the general public, as well as an adoption of increasing responsibility for communicating such events, I consider that it is important to remain vigilant about the fact that most abuse occurs at the hands of perpetrators who belong to the constellation of family members and friends, and that it may go uncovered until the survivors reach adulthood.

I should like to conclude this chapter by returning to Levey's (1999) paper on the role of the media in the area of child abuse. His valid comments about the feasibility of exploiting all aspects of the popular media in order to inform public opinion in the most enlightened, sensitive, and rounded manner, are worthy of serious note. He suggests that editors and broadcasters can be responsive to gentle pressure that promotes the educational, ethical, and empirical value of a proposed storyline. It is my opinion that in addition to providing a specialist service for survivors of CSA, we also have a duty to act as watchdogs concerning the types of popularly published material that could either help or hinder survivors, public opinion, and caring professionals.

Finally, I would be disloyal to a very sensitive and insightful reporter of the one and only local newspaper in the community in which I practice if I did not pay tribute to her, in the light of this chapter's critique. Taking a leaf out of Levey's paper, I approached this reporter and expressed my concern about recent publications that did not offer sufficiently rounded comment on the issue of CSA. Not only did the reporter acknowledge my concerns but agreed to interview me in order to dispel the myths surrounding the topic of CSA. The countless positive comments I subsequently received from survivors, expressing their relief at being able to read a realistic account of their experience, spoke for themselves.

Chapter 3

Definitions and prevalence of CSA

Academic interest and (in particular) empirical research in the field of child sexual abuse (CSA) are arguably still in their infancy. Granted, there are currently four major journals devoted exclusively to research on child abuse, which does reflect the growth of academic activity over the past two decades. However, empirical reviews seeking to evaluate the prevalence of CSA are a relatively recent phenomenon and consistent work in this area is sadly lacking where British population surveys are concerned. The purpose of this chapter is to provide a summary of our current state of knowledge, specifically in relation to issues regarding the problems encountered when attempting to define CSA, and also those relating to prevalence studies for both adults and children.

DEFINITIONS OF CSA

In the previous chapter I offered an overview of the changing attitudes in the popular media regarding child abuse in general and sexual abuse in particular, and in the final chapter I shall be addressing the crucial issue of society's responsibility towards the abuse of children. However, we must also remain vigilant to the historical and cultural double standards, variations, and inconsistencies that exist with regard to this very emotive topic.

In a review of the evidence on paedophilia, McConaghy (1998) offers some thought-provoking ideas on historical changes in the last century concerning adult/adolescent heterosexual behaviour. Similarly, Bullough (1990) points out examples suggesting not only that heterosexual behaviour between adults and adolescents has been tolerated during certain times throughout history, but that it has, in some instances, been the norm. One good example is the love affair between Romeo and Juliet, which, if it occurred today would be viewed as paedophilic, because Romeo is accepted by scholars as having been an adult while Juliet's age was thirteen years. Other examples quoted by Bullough are the sexual liaisons with minors of highly regarded figures such as the prophet Mohamed, Saint Augustine, and, more recently, Gandhi.

Further historical and cultural variations include the fact that in England until 1929 the legal age for marriage and sexual consent for girls was twelve (McConaghy, 1998), while in the USA it was, until recently, fourteen (Bullough, 1990). Currently, in New Zealand, The Netherlands, Spain, and Malta the age of heterosexual consent is twelve, while in Sweden, Poland, Denmark, the Czech Republic, France, and Greece it is fifteen (Government of the State of New South Wales, 1997). Bearing in mind these variations across time and between cultures, it is not surprising that there is no universally accepted definition of what constitutes child sexual abuse (Glaser and Frosh, 1993; Ferguson, 1997; Vogeltanz et al, 1999; Leventhal, 1998, 2000). This is understandable in view of the fact that such an act is a construction of a number of variables that may give rise to disagreement, controversy, and lack of clarity, not to mention differences in ideological, cultural, or ethical principles. If we look closely at the three stories set out in Chapter 2, we can elicit the following variables:

- age of the child;
- type of sexual act;
- nature of perpetrator; and
- absence of informed consent/coercion.

Taking these into account, it becomes clearer how a universally accepted definition of what constitutes sexual abuse can become problematic.

Let us take the issue of the age of the child. There is no generally accepted view, even among certain professionals, about when a child becomes "sexually mature" and the implication of this for "consent". Where is the demarcation? In certain cultures girls can marry as young as twelve or thirteen and start reproducing soon after. Certainly, we have all heard of cases that have gone to court in Western cultures where a judge may have deemed a child "sexually mature" or "provocative" in an attempt to atone for the acts of a defendant facing sexual abuse charges. An additional grey area relates to incest. While in legal or technical terms incest implies a blood relationship, as well as a penetrative act, for most professionals in the field incest is any sexual act imposed on a minor by any member of the family constellation.

There is also the difficulty of defining what "acts" constitute sexual abuse. Some definitions that I will discuss in a moment are, at best, partly inclusive of both contact as well as non-contact abuse, while others are too general and vague. This lack of clarity becomes particularly problematic when attempting to measure the extent of CSA, as will become evident when I address the issue of prevalence in the next section. Most researchers and, in particular, clinicians who work with survivors, however, agree that of utmost importance is the experience of being coerced into enduring or performing acts where the individual has no ability to provide informed consent; moreover these acts, whether or not they involve body contact, are employed by the perpetrator for the purpose of their own sexual gratification (e.g. Ferguson, 1997; McConaghy, 1998; Vogeltanz et al, 1999). Certainly, the experiences of CSA of the 180 women that will be addressed in the next chapter involved a wide range of sexually coercive acts by the perpetrators of their abuse, including penetrative acts, contact abuse over clothing, contact abuse under clothing, and non-contact abuse (for details, see Chapter 4).

In the UK, the 1988 Cleveland inquiry into the management of suspected victims of CSA proposed a working definition that read as follows: "The involvement of dependent, developmentally immature children and adolescents in sexual activities that they do not fully comprehend and to which they are unable to give informed consent or that violate the social taboos of family roles" (HMSO, 1988, p. 4). Although not very specific, this definition is flexible enough to include both contact and non-contact sexual acts, and most importantly, it raises the crucial issue of informed consent. Indeed, it is this latter point that has, in my opinion, the potential to override any conflicting views about what constitutes CSA.

I personally favour Sanderson's (1990) definitions because they are inclusive of most of the elements I have encountered in my own work, and also because they fulfil most of the criteria for a good working framework when studying sexual abuse. Her definitions are split into two categories— sexual abuse and incest. Sexual abuse is defined as:

> the involvement of dependent children and adolescents in sexual activities with an adult, or any person older or bigger, in which the child is used as a sexual object for the gratification of the older person's needs or desires, and to which the child is unable to give consent due to the unequal power in the relationship. This definition excludes consensual activity between peers.
>
> (Sanderson, 1990, p. 13)

The only qualification I would make to this definition is to add the word "informed" prior to "consent". In my experience, this is very important when treating adult survivors, because frequently they will blame themselves for accepting bribes from the perpetrator—such as money, gifts, or general favours—and assume that this made them accomplices in the sexual acts. During the course of therapy it becomes clear to them that this does not constitute informed consent because of the absence of adequate emotional, psychological, and cognitive development on their part at the time of the abuse, and that they would not have had the appropriate resources to form a decision or, indeed, to understand the implications of such an act.

Sanderson goes on to define incest as:

> a sexual act imposed on a child or adolescent by any person within the family constellation who abuses their position of power and trust within the family. It includes all sexual encounters where there is a difference of age and power, and all types of sexual behaviours ranging from pornography, voyeurism, exhibitionism, fondling, masturbation through to penile penetration. Most importantly, this definition includes all family members who have power over, and an investment of trust from, the child. To this effect it includes stepfathers, resident male friends of the family, uncles, brothers, grandfathers, cousins, as well as female relatives or family friends.
>
> (Sanderson, 1990, pp. 13–14)

These two definitions contain the main elements that I have encountered in my own experience of treating female survivors of sexual abuse. The inequality of the situation with its emphasis on the advantage of "power" in favour of the perpetrator; his/her psychological and/or physical coercion, and the exploitation of the child for the purpose of the perpetrator's sexual gratification, have appeared to be the primary elements in terms of the long-term psychological implications. In particular, the breach of trust, independent of whether the perpetrator was a blood relation or not, have seemed to be a crucial factor in the development of negative long-term effects. These factors will be discussed in greater detail in Chapter 5.

PREVALENCE

The previous section highlighted the difficulties inherent in defining sexual abuse, and the reasons for this were discussed. Equally problematic is the area of categorising the various acts that are considered to constitute sexual abuse. Given these complexities, the issue of prevalence becomes an additional challenge to those who attempt to measure the frequency of CSA because the collection and analyses of data will vary according to the individual's operational definition. In addition, there is of course the issue of the different types of methodology adopted when surveying the extent of CSA, which has also been considered to be a cause of biases in prevalence variability (Gorey and Leslie, 1997; Leventhal, 2000). Equally crucial is the recognition that where adult disclosure of sexual abuse is concerned, we only know of those who come forward and, therefore, samples are inevitably self-selected. Issues such as shame, self-blame, and fear of not being believed are very powerful factors in deterring people from disclosing their abuse. Certainly, in my own experience, most women I talked to did not disclose the abuse until they were adults, while most of those who "told" were either not believed or were reprimanded for doing so, therefore, reinforcing their silence. Certainly, the growing awareness of the existence of sexual abuse, which has led to media interest, has encouraged an increase in those who currently come forward, and we may see a resulting change in figures relating to incidence (the number of new sexual abuse cases in the population) as well as prevalence (how much sexual abuse exists).

The existing research includes figures based on the retrospective disclosure of adults, those based on the disclosure by children, and those based on cases that are uncovered by professionals involved with them (e.g. social services, therapeutic agencies, the police, etc.).

Adults

It is important to gain an appreciation of the perspective afforded by the rather brief history of empirical studies that have sought to evaluate the prevalence of CSA. A few of the "classic" surveys in the adult population, which are frequently mentioned, deserve some attention. For example, Baker and Duncan (1985) carried out one of the largest studies in Britain involving a nationally representative sample of 2,019 women and men, using a definition which stipulated that a child is involved with a sexually mature person in "any activity which the other person expects to lead to their sexual arousal" (Baker and Duncan, 1985, p. 459). The activities included in their definition involved intercourse as well as all contact and non-contact activities. The results of their study suggested that 12 per cent of women and 8 per cent of men had been abused before the age of sixteen. The suggestion in this study, however, that female sexual abuse is more common for women than for men may be misleading due to the lower incidence of reporting in men, because of the argument that males find it more difficult to disclose their abuse experience (Finkelhor, 1984). Another study in Britain (Hall, 1985) suggested that 21 per cent of a sample of 1,236 women reported being abused as children, while 600 women surveyed by West (1985) revealed that 46 per cent of them recalled being sexually abused in their childhood.

Sadly, as mentioned earlier, there exists a dearth in population surveys of the extent of CSA in the UK. The most recent review of such work that I was able to find was Ferguson (1997), who concluded that there continued to exist much debate about the true frequency of CSA. Although this review was written in 1997, the quoted figure of 10 per cent relating to the estimated prevalence of CSA made use of the Baker and Duncan (1985) study mentioned in the previous paragraph. Unfortunately, not much progress has been made since, despite Ferguson's concluding remarks appealing for further refined and updated epidemiological studies of CSA, together with a call for a standardisation of definitions and employment of outcome measures for future studies of both the frequency and long-term effects of CSA. Such studies in the UK continue to be urgently awaited.

Elsewhere, varying prevalence rates of CSA have been found. Most empirical research in this area since the mid-1980s has taken place in North America, and one of the first classic studies was that of Finkelhor (1984). He suggested that between 12 per cent and 38 per cent of women were sexually abused as children, while the figure for men was between 2.5 and 9 per cent. Another study by Lewis (1985), based on a random sample of the population of the entire USA, was carried out using half-hour telephone interviews with 1,374 females. Based on a broad definition of sexual abuse, the results showed that 27 per cent of the women reported sexual abuse in childhood. Around the same time, the classic and frequently quoted studies of Wyatt and Peters (1986a, 1986b) concerned themselves with issues of CSA relating to definition, prevalence, and methodology. Bearing in mind that they were smaller community studies, Wyatt and Peters (1986a) reported that 53 per cent of a random sample of 131 women in Los Angeles were sexually abused as children, while Russell's (1983) study based in San Francisco reported that 54 per cent were abused, based on a random sample of 594 women.

Finkelhor (1994a) undertook the challenge of reviewing child abuse from an international perspective, using 21 epidemiological studies of child abuse in non-clinical populations of adults from at least nineteen countries. Abuse rates were comparable to those of North America, with figures ranging from 7 to 36 per cent for women and from 3 to 29 per cent for men, confirming that sexual abuse is an international problem. In line with international figures, a large study conducted by Anderson et al (1993) in New Zealand found that, based on a response rate of 73 per cent of women under the age of sixty-five (the total random sample targeted consisted of 3,000 women), nearly one woman in three reported having one or more unwanted sexual experience before the age of sixteen. Some 70 per cent of these cases involved genital contact or more severe abuse, and 12 per cent of those abused were subjected to sexual intercourse.

As I mentioned at the start of this chapter, recent population surveys on the prevalence of CSA appear to be lacking and I was only able to find very few such studies. Of interest is Wyatt et al's (1999) update of Wyatt's (1985) study in Los Angeles, which targeted African and European American women aged between eighteen and fifty, and sought to compare current figures and circumstances to those reported in the previous decade. The sample was obtained through random digit telephone dialling procedures, and each of the 338 participants who took part in the survey were interviewed face-to-face by a trained interviewer of the same ethnicity. The results of this study suggested that there were no significant changes in the overall prevalence of CSA compared with the previous decade; equally, there were no significant differences in the prevalence figures between ethnic groups. That is, 34 per cent of the total sample reported at least one incident of CSA prior to age eighteen, while 40 per cent of the women reported more than one incident, making the figures comparable to those reported in 1985. Another recent study by Vogeltanz et al (1999) targeting a large North American population of 1,099 women found CSA prevalence rates to be consistent with Finkelhor's (1994b) estimate of 20 per cent or higher. In the Vogeltanz et al survey, the estimated prevalence, taking into account the two definitions of CSA that they employed, was 17.3–24 per cent.

In attempting to summarise the overall state of knowledge relating to prevalence of CSA, my search for up-to-date reviews of the current picture, unfortunately, did not shed more light on the above summary of some of the classic studies, possibly due to the apparent slowing down of activity in this area. Indeed, the more recent reviews on the subject I was able to find (e.g. Ferguson, 1997; Leventhal, 1998; Fleming, 1998) made use of the figures from older surveys such as the ones that I have just discussed, including one study in Ontario (Macmillan et al, 1997) which reported that the prevalence rate of CSA in the general population was 12.8 per cent for women and 4.3 per cent for men. Taking what is known to date into account, the reviews summarise the reported prevalence of CSA as varying from 6 to 62 per cent for women and 3 to 39 per cent for men.

An informative paper by Gorey and Leslie (1997) reviewed the effects of methodological variations on reported CSA prevalence rates for non-clinical samples. The authors argued that child abuse definitions and response rates accounted for half of the observed variability of the reported prevalence rates. Further, their review concluded that when greater response rates were observed in studies, the prevalence estimate of CSA was lower. Adjusting for these effects, Gorey and Leslie argued that the true prevalence of CSA fell somewhere between 12 and 17 per cent for women and 5 and 8 per cent for men. Although the authors called for large, methodologically rigorous, population-based studies, they made the relevant and crucial point that having established beyond doubt that CSA does occur and is widespread, what is urgently needed is more research and investigation into the long-term effects of CSA, as well as methods for prevention. The latter observation could not have been more insightful and encouraging, as evidenced by the recent flurry of academic activity concerning the long-term effects of CSA as well as child protection (see Chapter 5). Consequently, the current dearth of population surveys is at least partly understandable, and the observation that Gorey and Leslie's appeal for more work in the area of long-term effects has been answered is very gratifying.

Clinical populations

Controlled studies of the prevalence of CSA in clinical populations are neither abundant nor conclusive. Once again, recent reviews make use of historical "classic" studies in this area and there continues to be an urgent need for a more up-to-date picture of the current state of affairs. One frequently quoted study is that of Bryer et al (1987), which looked at sixty-six female psychiatric in-patients and reported that 21 per cent had experienced sexual abuse alone, while 59 per cent had experienced both sexual and physical abuse. Other studies in the USA have included Herman's (1986) research, which found that in a sample of 105 psychiatric outpatient women, 13 per cent reported CSA. In Miller et al's (1993) study focusing on women being treated for alcohol problems, 70 per cent reported having been sexually abused in childhood. A more recent study (Coverdale and Turbott, 2000) compared the extent of sexual and physical abuse of 158 chronically ill psychiatric outpatients of both genders with matched controls who had never been treated for psychiatric illness. Although there were no significant differences in the rates of sexual and physical abuse in childhood (28.5 per cent and 27.3 per cent, respectively) between patients and controls, psychiatric patients—and in particular women—were more likely to have experienced sexual and physical abuse in adulthood, especially when CSA had occurred, than controls. Given these results, the authors called for psychiatrists to routinely enquire about abuse experiences.

British studies have included that of Metcalfe (1994) which took place in Leicester and sought to estimate the prevalence of CSA in a group of patients suffering from eating disorders, and a group of general psychiatric outpatients. Unfortunately this was not a very well-controlled study as it employed a group of GP patients as controls. The results indicated that 32 per cent of the eating disorders' group, 49 per cent of the female psychiatric outpatients, and 23 per cent of the male psychiatric outpatients had experienced sexual abuse in childhood. Of those attending GP surgeries, 46 per cent of female and 14 per cent of male patients reported a history of CSA, but it was recognised that a more representative sample of the general population would provide a better comparison in future studies.

Ferguson (1997) points out that studies of the prevalence of CSA in clinical populations are subject to the same methodological difficulties as those of non-clinical samples. A further important point is made concerning the controversy relating to the possibility of false memory syndrome among patients who are receiving therapy. This sensitive and topical issue will be addressed in detail in Chapter 14, with particular reference to my own experience of treating hundreds of women with histories of CSA. Suffice it to say that the false/recovered memory debate has been of little relevance to my work as a therapist, and this issue will also be discussed in Chapter 14.

In Chapter 4 I discuss the descriptive variables that define the group of 180 women whom I have focused on in the course of writing this book, and the reader will be able to gain a good impression of the relevant issues that survivors have discussed, such as the nature of perpetrator as well as the type, frequency, and duration of abuse. While it was not my intention to provide a controlled comparison of the prevalence of CSA, I have found it interesting to note that of a total of about 2,500 patients seen to date (mostly women), approximately 17 per cent have disclosed an experience of CSA. This figure is compatible with the lower rates of prevalence noted in the general population and highlights the need for more well-controlled studies and surveys in the clinical and general populations.

Children and adolescents

It is now well acknowledged that not only do children find it difficult to tell anyone that they are being sexually abused (Leventhal 2000; Edgarth and Ormstad 2000), but also that disclosure of sexual abuse to parents and professionals is more likely to occur in adulthood rather than in childhood. This makes the measuring of the true incidence of sexual abuse very difficult to assess, and raises the critical issue of lack of prompt intervention. One good example of such delay is the study of Smith et al (2000), who gathered representative data regarding the length of time prior to disclosing pre-age eighteen rape in a sample of 3,200 women. Some 28 per cent of child rape victims reported that they had never told anyone about their experience prior to the research interview, while for 47 per cent of the sample it was five years following the experience before they disclosed it, with close friends being the most common confidants. When the perpetrator was a "stranger" the delay in disclosure was shorter, whereas three factors—if the perpetrator was a family member, repeated assaults, and younger age of the victim—were associated with longer delays in telling anyone.

In addition to the delay in disclosing abuse, another problem is whether it is ethical or feasible to ask children direct questions about their experiences of sexual abuse. Although clinicians do ask children about such occurrences in appropriate clinical settings, few studies have sought to gather data directly from children, or even adolescents. Some of the concerns regarding such studies have related to the necessity of providing safety for the children who disclose abuse and to the involvement of child protection services. In addition, there has been the concern about children's ability to understand the questions asked of them and also the accuracy of children's reports (Leventhal, 2000). Although there is a dearth of studies that have attempted to overcome these difficulties, two are worthy of mention. The first is that of Finkelhor and Dziuba-Leatherman (1994), which was the first to report on a telephone survey of children that focused specifically on victimisation. Steps taken to protect the minors included obtaining consent for the interview from both parent and child, ensuring that the child was alone and free to speak, offering the telephone number of a national helpline, and provision of professional help if there was concern about current harm. The survey targeted 2,000 children aged between ten and sixteen who were selected from a nationally representative sample and interviewed over the telephone. Of this total, 10.5 per cent reported having experienced sexual abuse, with a further 6.7 per cent reporting such abuse in the previous year.

A more recent Swedish study, Edgarth and Ormstad (2000), targeted 1,943 17-year-old students and 210 school-leavers of the same age. Subjects completed self-administered anonymous questionnaires that were distributed by school nurses. The questions asked dealt with personal experiences of sexual abuse, including age at onset; frequency; and relationship to perpetrator. The definition used excluded sexual experiences with peers. Among the male and female students, 3.1 per cent and 11.2 per cent, respectively, said that they had experienced sexual abuse, while among the school non-attenders, 4 per cent of the boys and 28 per cent of the girls, respectively, admitted to experiencing sexual abuse. An important issue raised by the authors of this study is that, overall, very few of the adolescents had disclosed their abuse to a professional.

In Britain, as far as I have been able to ascertain, no surveys on the prevalence or incidence of sexual abuse have targeted children directly. Some figures from varying sources, however, have provided, across time, an interesting if not very consistent picture. For example, Mrazek et al (1983) targeted 1,599 professionals such as paediatricians, general practitioners, police surgeons, and child psychiatrists, finding that sexual abuse in children was uncovered in 1,072 cases in the year 1977–78. This figure was argued at the time to represent one child in 6,000. Glacer and Frosh (1993), however, argued that it may have been a gross underestimation of the true incidence of sexual abuse in children due to methodological problems in the study. For example, the overall response rate from the professionals contacted was 39 per cent, with only 16 per cent of the general practitioners returning their forms. A further problem was that the study was restricted to cases that had been identified via the formal professional channels, and it was argued that, "at every stage, from disclosure by a child to response by a professional to registration as a statistic, there are reasons why sexual abuse is neglected and overlooked" (Glacer and Frosh, 1993, p. 10). Seven years after Mrazek et al's (1983) statistics, the NSPCC (1990) produced an estimate of the national incidence of sexual abuse in England and Wales, based on the number of children who were registered with them. For children under the ages of fourteen and sixteen, 5,850 and 6,600, respectively, had been sexually abused, and, of these, 78 per cent were girls and 22 per cent were boys. To complicate matters further, the Department of Health (1993) revealed that the overall rate of CSA registrations in 1992 comprised 24 per cent girls and 11 per cent boys. Ferguson (1997), however, rightfully argues that the problem with such statistics is that they only refer to cases of CSA that have been detected by professionals and/or those that have been reported voluntarily.

In ending this discussion on the prevalence/incidence of CSA in children and adolescents, it is important to quote the very recent figures published by ChildLine (2000). In the year 1997–98 they counselled over 115,000 children, of which 20 per cent telephoned about physical abuse, sexual abuse, or both. Although the present discussion on the prevalence of CSA among children and adolescents has not been an exhaustive one, the findings mentioned clearly highlight not only that we are far from knowing the true incidence of CSA but also that further work in this area is urgently needed.

CONCLUSIONS

This second part of this chapter has attempted to provide a summary of the main findings in the area of prevalence/incidence of CSA for adults, children, and adolescents. An historical perspective of the more frequently quoted pieces of work has been discussed, as well as an overview of the current state of affairs. There is no doubt that in the past two decades our knowledge in this very difficult area of investigation has increased, while, at the same time, what we currently know points to the need for further and better controlled and methodologically sound studies. It is true that as our awareness of the extent of the prevalence of CSA has grown, so has the work in this complex area sought to diversify its attention to allied crucial concerns, such as the consequences of CSA, the issue of child protection, and of course the psychology and management of perpetrators. Each of these issues will be addressed in detail in subsequent chapters, but it is important to conclude this chapter by pointing out some important issues that require attention in future empirical work. Leventhal (1998) has summarised some of these areas and has called for the following: additional surveys on the prevalence of CSA in men; studies on the effects of different methodologies in the elicitation of past sexual abuse; prevalence studies of CSA in developing countries; surveys of the prevalence of CSA using national probability samples of adults; and finally, taking into account the fact that the rate of disclosure of sexual abuse to relevant authorities (e.g. the police and child protection services) has been low, it would be useful to carry out surveys that might compare the current rate of such disclosure given the increase in societal and professional awareness as well as recognition of CSA.

Chapter 4

The survivors: Summary of descriptive variables in a group of women who were sexually abused as children

INTRODUCTION

In Chapter 1 I explained how the idea and purpose for this book were generated and I emphasised the long-standing nature of its development. In this chapter I present a breakdown of variables that have been gathered over several years during the course of my clinical work with survivors. In Chapter 1 I also made clear that the statistical material presented in this book is essentially descriptive and explained why no standardised data—i.e. questionnaires or formal assessment measures—were used to elicit the variables. The latter have been gathered and recorded following a very lengthy and painstaking exercise involving the meticulous examination of each individual personal file. I hope that presenting a summary of the variables (based on a total of 180 women) that I consider to be pertinent to gaining an overall view of the survivors' background will achieve the following:

- It will familiarise the reader with the group of women I have worked with.
- It may contribute to a clearer appreciation of the issues that will be addressed in the intervention chapter.
- It may offer readers the opportunity, if they so wish, of making their own comparisons with other published material (i.e. with reference to some of the variables relating to sexual abuse).
- It may provide those who are not very familiar with some of the facets of sexual abuse—such as the nature of perpetrators, types of sexual abuse, and so on—with an "extended snapshot" of such variables and their frequency within a clinical population.

Before I present the summary of the variables, it may also be of benefit to describe, briefly, the community within which I work. I consider this to be important not only because this community, I believe, has some unique features, but also because by describing it I will be completing the picture of the setting in which this book was written. My initial clinical work follow-ing my training (in the late 1980s) was carried out in two major teaching hospitals in London, and these had relatively large as well as heterogeneous catchment areas. Although my involvement with female survivors of child sexual abuse (CSA) dates since that period, this involvement truly inten-sified and developed during the course of my work in the community in which I have been living and practising since the early 1990s. I am employed in one of the Channel Islands as a member of the only clinical psychology department (equivalent to clinical psychology departments in the NHS on the mainland), due to the island's small population (less than 90,000).

On starting my employment I made it known that I had a special interest in working with female survivors of sexual abuse and it may be that this announcement had a bearing on the fact that the number of women referred for this reason increased steadily over the initial period of my work in the community. Although there are other practitioners who are in private practice, as well as voluntary agencies that provide a service for survivors, as indeed do some of my colleagues, in such a small island "word of mouth" has a way of circulating information and making people, in various professional areas, become very quickly known and assimilated at the heart of the community. A senior member of our social services department once commented at a local conference: "When the rafts are brought out, that is when people come forward for rescuing". He was not referring to sexual abuse, in particular, but his words seem to reflect what may have occurred when I arrived in this community.

Another aspect of working in a small community is that while "word of mouth" can be positive, it can also be very negative and have serious implications for anyone that is not seen to be "delivering the goods". This state of affairs can potentially cause a certain degree of discomfort if it is perceived as having one's actions being subjected to microscopic scrutiny. In my case, however, I have experienced this situation as an adjunct to the professional conscience I adhere to, and I will discuss this later when I present a section on the therapeutic relationship. I believe that being accountable in such an obvious manner can actually have a positive influence on one's professional ethics. First of all, there is continuous feedback, be it good or bad, and if this is utilised constructively it can offer invaluable professional guidance. Secondly, working in this close-knit environment has proved to be most satisfying in terms of my clinical involvement because, on the one hand, the island is far too small for migration to occur and, therefore, it is quite common for patients to return for completion of their therapy. On the other hand, there is a continuous population movement, of young people in particular, and this means that there is always the possibility for newcomers to present for therapy. On a personal level, I have always found it heart-warming when, inevitably, my path crosses with those of survivors, and even long after their therapy has been completed, they appear to be at ease about filling me in on some aspects of their lives.

I appreciate that these descriptions may be appealing to some, but not to other professionals who are practising psychotherapists and who may prefer to keep a clear boundary between their work and their private lives. In my case, my initial trepidation very quickly gave way to great professional satisfaction and, indeed, the impetus for writing this book is founded in the setting in which I work. Now that the "scene" has been set for the material that will follow, it is appropriate here to make some observations about the variables that will be presented.

The first and most important observation to bear in mind is that although the therapeutic work was carried out in the community I have just described, that community is nevertheless an extremely heterogeneous one in that the ratio of local population to migrants from the mainland is continuously fluctuating and the latter have been known to exceed the former. In addition, there is a significant minority of people who have come to the island either as children or adults from a number of other European countries, and there are a few who have come from other continents. Certainly, the women I see and the group I am referring to in this book have diverse origins and, therefore, no distinction is being made in relation to place of origin. Secondly, the variables presented are not based on any a priori assumptions, because the book is the result of a gradual progression based, essentially, on therapeutic work with female survivors. Moreover, I have deliberately avoided the "objectification" of the women's experience through the use of standardised questionnaires, and the information presented is based on a painstaking and thorough review of my notes on the women's individual histories. It may be argued, therefore, that the variables I have included are arbitrary, and also, that there could be many others which I have omitted. However, the ones presented reflect recurring themes across all the survivors and this, therefore, reinforces the view that while there are common themes expressed by survivors of sexual abuse, their experience is nevertheless subjective, and I considered that it would be essential to observe both these aspects.

Overall, the variables presented can be very broadly categorised in terms of being "person specific", "abuse specific", and "other relevant variables". The first includes basic demographic information, such as age at referral, marital status, and so on, which may help the reader to become acquainted with the survivors and also with the agency they were referred from. The second category refers to variables that are specifically related to the history and experience of sexual abuse, and the ones presented reflect the areas that are of most concern to the survivors. The third category refers to variables perceived by survivors as pertinent in terms of relevance to their experience of sexual abuse and, for some, these include issues such as making formal statements to the police and the outcome of such actions. Variables related to other issues raised at initial presentation for therapy, such as excessive use of alcohol, use of illicit drugs, and self-harm, are also included in this category, as well as a subjective "global rating", referring to the degree of "coping" with daily life at initial presentation for therapy. More detailed discussion on the subject of psychological, emotional, and behavioural consequences are accorded individual attention in Chapter 5.

THE VARIABLES

"Person specific" variables

Age at referral

Table 4.1 summarises the frequency of women's age at the time of referral.[1] It shows that the age range of women who were referred was sixteen to fifty-nine and that almost half of the women were between the ages of twenty and twenty-nine, followed by another quarter of women who were between the ages of thirty and thirty-nine.

Table 4.1   Women's ages at time of referral

Age range	Frequency	Percentage
16–19	13	7.2
20–29	89	49.4
30–39	46	25.6
40–49	26	14.4
50–59	6	3.3
Total	180	100.0

It would be interesting to have further information about what these frequencies suggest. Some considerations may relate to the following. First, whether age has any bearing on the wish to seek help and, if so, why. Secondly, whether the fact that the smallest age range at referral—i.e. fifty to fifty-nine—suggests either positive adaptation and/or resolution of the experience of sexual abuse, or that women in that age range might feel reluctant for a number of reasons to present for therapy. Thirdly, whether the fact that only 7 per cent of the women referred were between the ages of sixteen and nineteen might suggest that either more women in this age group are being treated in child and family units, or that (as I would be likely to speculate) women in this age range are still relatively young and may not have yet encountered the types of life events that have a tendency to bring memories of sexual abuse to the surface. I would further argue that the "denial" stage that can follow the experience of sexual abuse can remain in some individuals well into their teens and twenties, and in some others for an indefinite period.

Referral source

Table 4.2 summarises the frequency of the various referral sources. It shows that just over half of the women I saw (51 per cent) were referred by their general practitioners. The next two highest referral sources were psychiatry (15 per cent) and the women who referred themselves (11.7 per cent). The rest of the referrals came from a variety of sources that included social services; child/family service; the police; voluntary services (i.e. Women's Refuge; Rape Crisis; Relate; Hospice); non-psychiatric medical and nursing staff; and "other" (i.e. educational establishments and other therapists in private practice).

Table 4.2   Referral source

Source	Frequency	Percentage
GPs	92	51.1
Psychiatry	27	15.0
Self	21	11.7
Voluntary services	13	7.2
Social/child and family services	11	6.1
Medical doctors/nurses	7	3.9
Other	3	1.7
Total	**180**	**100.0**

Presenting problem

Table 4.3 shows the frequency of women who were referred for sexual abuse and also of those women whose initial referral did not mention the issue of such abuse.

Table 4.3   Presenting problem

Problem	Frequency	Percentage
Sexual abuse	157	87.2
Other	23	12.8
Total	**180**	**100.0**

There are some points requiring clarification regarding the information in this table. First, although the vast majority of the women (87 per cent) appear to have been referred for sexual abuse, most of these referral requests mentioned a combination with one or more of the following difficulties: depression, sexual difficulties, anxiety (particularly social anxiety), marital difficulties, "general dysphoria", relationship problems, self-harm, and addiction (i.e. alcohol and/or illicit drugs). The 12.8 per cent of women who were referred for "other" problems involved requests mentioning one or more of the difficulties listed above. The fact that I have not presented specific data regarding the individual cluster of presenting problems is intentional because I am not conducting an epidemiological study, and also because during the course of my work I have observed that referral letters do not always reflect an accurate picture of the problem when compared with the survivors' own subjective experience. Since it is the latter that is focused on here, it is the women's own perception of their general adaptation and difficulties that will be discussed later in this chapter.

Secondly, the reason I have included the information in Table 4.3 is in order to highlight the fact that, for the most part, I was not the first person to whom the experience of sexual abuse was disclosed. Indeed, only 23 women of the total number I saw for sexual abuse said that they had never disclosed the fact to a professional before, and these were mostly the women who were self-referred. An observation worth making here is that it appears as though women may be less reluctant to come forward and talk about their experience and also to seek help.

Thirdly, Table 4.3 may reassure those who may fear that the "disclosure" of sexual abuse can be a function of certain therapeutic techniques (e.g. hypnosis). This relates to some of the controversies that have arisen in the 1990s, both in the therapeutic field and also the legal arena, concerning the validity of some disclosures of sexual abuse. I am referring here to the concepts of "false memory syndrome" and "recovered memory", and I consider this an important enough issue to accord it particular attention in Chapter 14, in which I will discuss some of the literature on the subject and will refer to specific instances in my own clinical work (which have been very few indeed) when the "disclosure" of sexual abuse was doubtful. Suffice it to say that, where all 180 women are concerned here, it is my professional and personal belief that their disclosures are totally genuine and that I do not use hypnosis or "auto-suggestive" manipulation in my work.

Marital status and children

Table 4.4 shows the distribution of the type of relationship status of the women at the time of referral, while Table 4.5 shows the number of women with children.

Table 4.4 indicates that the majority of the women were in some form of relationship at the time they presented for therapy. Those who had boyfriends did not live with them and most of those with partners had been in the relationship for some time. The breakdown of the various categories is not in itself remarkable and the only speculation I would make here is that

Table 4.4   Marital status

Status	Frequency	Percentage
Married	61	33.9
Single	57	31.7
Partner	32	17.8
Divorced	16	8.9
Boyfriend	11	6.1
No data	3	1.7
Total	**180**	**100.0**

Table 4.5   Frequency and percentage of women with children

Children	Frequency	Percentage
Yes	89	49.4
No	84	46.7
No data	7	3.9
Total	**180**	**100.0**

the fact that just over half the women were in stable relationships and most had children (see Table 4.5) may have created the "right" conditions for seeking help. Two such conditions spring to mind: one is that they felt they had a sufficiently stable base from which to address past or current problems, and the second is that actually being faced with difficulties in their current life (e.g. difficult relationships and/or child rearing) triggered hitherto unresolved or unprocessed emotional issues. The women in general gave different reasons for seeking help, but it was common for those women with children to say that either they were afraid of abusing their children because they had been abused (and had "heard" or "read" accounts about this connection) and, therefore, they wished to address their own abuse, or that actually being involved with their children was bringing up memories of their own childhood which they had "pushed to the back of their minds". In many other cases it was the interpersonal and sexual aspects of their relationships with their partners that acted as an impetus to seeking help. Interestingly, the single and divorced group of women also stated that either the lack of a relationship, or the choice of "wrong" or unsuitable partners was an important factor for seeking help. These issues will be discussed further later in this chapter.

Foster care/residential home

The number of women who reported having experienced periods in foster care, residential homes, or both was very small. Overall, nine women said they had been in foster care for some periods during their childhood; nine women said they had the experience of being in intermittent residential care; and only three women said they had experience of both. Some revealed that their sexual abuse occurred in one of these circumstances and this will be discussed when the distribution of perpetrators is presented. I would like to remind readers that because the women's origins encompass a wide variety of geographical locations, so too do their childhood histories.

Concluding thoughts on "person specific" variables

I am aware that I could have included other relevant information under this heading, such as educational and also employment history, as well as information relating to the families of the women, but I decided not to for two reasons. First, in relation to the issue of family background when sexual abuse or incest occurs, this is too complex to be simply reduced to a "figures" discussion. The many variables and dynamics within the family are far too important and require an in-depth discussion, and this will be accorded separate attention later in the book. Issues such as domestic violence, alcoholism, psychological abuse, neglect, instability of parental relationships, and so on are all interdependent and an attempt at separating them is, in my view, too simplistic. Indeed, what was confirmed to me by the survivors of sexual abuse is that the family or home background within which the abuse occurred had, at times, a greater impact on the survivors in terms of their emotional and psychological difficulties.

The second reason for avoiding a reductionist approach with respect to socio-economic and educational factors is that my experience working on sexual abuse cases has more than confirmed that its existence observes no cultural, educational, or economic differences. Equally, with respect to the women themselves, it is their psychological and emotional characteristics I wish to focus on. Also, personal growth is, in my opinion, potentially independent of socio-economic constraints.

"Abuse specific" variables

Perpetrator

Table 4.6 provides data on the frequency of each type of perpetrator. It shows that in 80 per cent of the sexual abuse incidents the perpetrator was known to the woman, and that in 67 per cent the perpetrator was a blood relative or close member of the family, with natural fathers accounting for a third (33 per cent) of the incidents of abuse and stepfathers for 17 per cent. With the exception of three incidents of sexual abuse by the mother, all the perpetrators were male. Only three women identified their biological mothers as being the perpetrator of the abuse, and therefore accounted for just under 2 per cent of the whole group of women seen.

Table 4.6   Perpetrator

Perpetrator	Frequency	Percentage
Father	59	32.8
Stepfather/partner (mother's)	31	17.2
Uncle	19	10.6
Brother	14	7.8
Grandfather	8	4.4
Friend of family	8	4.4
Neighbour	8	4.4
Brother-in-law	6	3.3
Stranger	5	2.8
Mother	3	1.7
Cousin	2	1.1
Other	9	5.0
No data	8	4.4
Total	**180**	**100.0**

The category of abusers under the title of "stranger" in Table 4.6 was so named to indicate that the perpetrator was neither familiar nor known to the survivor. The five strangers identified here perpetuated the abuse on one occasion only and the survivors' perception of the abuse, as recounted in adult terms, constituted either an "assault" or "attack" and the form of abuse was anything from exhibitionism to actual rape. The fact that only five survivors of the 180 disclosed such abuse adds further credence to the notion that most abusers are known to survivors.

The category of "other" in Table 4.6 refers to teachers, care workers in residential institutions, and foster parents. This group accounts for 5 per cent of the total figure for abusers.[2]

A factor that needs addressing prior to concluding the discussion of the information in Table 4.6 is multiple abuse. Eighteen women from the group said that they had been abused by more than one perpetrator, and the one given priority for the sake of the category breakdown is the perpetrator the survivor perceived as having had the greatest negative impact on her. For example, if a woman was abused by her father and then another time by her uncle or brother, she would point to one of those as being the most damaging and he would, therefore, be the one entered in the table.

Age abuse started

Table 4.7 sets out the distribution of ages when the abuse started. The table indicates that nearly 34 per cent of the women said that their abuse started between the ages of five and seven. If this is combined with the range of eight to ten years of age, it implies that for 58 per cent of this group of women the abuse started when they were aged between five and ten. Just

Table 4.7 Women's age when abuse started

Age (in years)	Frequency	Percentage
2–4	15	8.3
5–7	61	33.9
8–10	44	24.4
11–14	44	24.4
No data	16	8.9
Total	**180**	**100.0**

under a quarter of the women said that their abuse started between the ages of eleven and fourteen, while 8 per cent said it started when they were aged between two and four. As previously noted, the missing values refer to the situation where survivors could not remember, or where they either did not pursue therapy or left therapy prior to disclosing such information.

The issue of age at the onset of CSA has not, in my experience, proved to be a reliable predictor of long-term effects, although in a study by Baker and Duncan (1985) there was a suggestion that women reporting most perceived ill-effects were abused before the age of ten. The issue of long-term effects will be introduced in the closing section of this chapter and will be the subject of detailed discussion in Chapter 5. The reason I have included this table is to make clear that sexual abuse can occur at almost any age.

Nature of abuse

For the purpose of clarity and manageability in categorising the frequencies of the different types of abuse in the group of women (see Table 4.8), I have used the following definitions:

- "I" stands for all acts that involve penetrative abuse involving the penis, finger, and objects; and also anal penetration.
- "C1" represents all contact abuse such as genital touching and fondling (mutual or otherwise); oral sex (receptive and/or given); and all acts of fondling and touching carried out on the naked body of the child/adolescent and perpetrator.
- "C2" represents all acts of touching (genital and/or non-genital) on the clothed body; and inappropriate kissing.
- "NC" includes all non-contact acts, comprising voyeurism; exhibitionism; verbal innuendo and/or sexual insults; showing pornography; inappropriate photography (i.e. taking exploitative photographs of the child for sexual gratification); disrespect of personal boundaries; and verbal requests of a sexual nature.

Table 4.8   Nature of abuse

Category	Frequency	Percentage
I	44	24.4
C1	87	48.3
C2	19	10.6
NC	3	1.7
No data	27	15.0
Total	**180**	**100.0**

Table 4.8 shows that just under half of the women described sexual abuse involving the more serious type of contact abuse, with another quarter (approximately) reporting abuse of the most intrusive kind involving some form of penetrative act on them. Some 10 per cent reported contact abuse of a less intrusive nature.

Although the table shows a breakdown of discrete categories of abuse, the picture presented by survivors is not that simple and an explanation is required. If we assume that the categories are ordered in terms of their severity, starting from the first (i.e. penetrative abuse), then most of the women would relate experiences of abuse in one or more of the lower categories also, and similarly for the next category (C1), and so on. In the reverse direction, however, the survivor would have only experienced the abuse shown. For example, a woman having experienced non-contact abuse (NC) would not have experienced abuse in any other form.

Duration of abuse

Table 4.9 gives a breakdown of the distribution of duration of abuse. The issue of duration of abuse was one that the majority of the women found difficult to be exact about, although for most the margin did not exceed approximately fifteen months. Those who were abused on only one occasion were the most confident about the accuracy of this, closely followed by the twenty women whose abuse did not exceed a period of one year. The rest of the table is self-explanatory and the only thing to add here is that, clearly, sexual abuse can occur only once, or, at the other extreme, persist for up to fifteen years. Here, the average duration of abuse for survivors would appear to be approximately five years and this seems to be compatible with other clinicians' reports (Courtois, 1988). However, it should be noted that this, as well as the other areas discussed in this chapter, are very personal to survivors and we only have what they are able to, or wish to tell us. Therefore, it is unwise to make gross generalisations other than to note that the duration of sexual abuse can be anything from very brief to very enduring and persistent.

Table 4.9   Duration of abuse

In years	Frequency	Percentage
Once	19	10.6
Up to 1 year	20	11.1
2–3	35	19.4
4–5	25	13.9
6–7	19	10.6
8–9	15	8.3
10–11	7	3.9
12–13	8	4.4
14–15	3	1.7
No data	29	16.1
Total	**180**	**100.0**

Frequency of abuse

This was another factor that survivors found difficult to estimate precisely. Ninety women (44 per cent) were either uncertain about the frequency of the abuse or did not offer such information. Of the rest, 55 women (31 per cent) said that the abuse was "frequent" in that it occurred at least on a weekly basis, 27 women (15 per cent) said that it was only "occasional", and 19 women (11 per cent) said that it occurred only once (as stated above). I am not able to give an explanation of this variable with any certainty, other than to speculate that children have a good capacity for denying or "locking away" very disturbing events or events that they are not able to comprehend. Consequently, it makes reasonable sense to assume that the survivors simply do not remember with accuracy the frequency of their abusive experiences. This issue will be discussed in more detail in Chapter 13 on "false" as well as "recovered" memory.

Other relevant variables

Police/court/conviction

Of the total of 180 women, 33 (18 per cent) had either made formal written statements against their perpetrator to the police at adulthood or were in the process of making such a statement during the course of their therapy and expected further action to be taken. Of these 33 cases taken to the police, 18 (10 per cent) culminated in legal proceedings involving a court case, with only 12 of the perpetrators (6.5 per cent) being convicted. Of the remaining women, 145 (80 per cent) said they had not made such complaints and did not wish to do so, and there is no data for two of the women.

I have included information on this variable because I have found that the issue of bringing sexual abuse to the attention of legal authorities has a significant role to play for those who decide to take up such action. The impact and ramifications resulting from survivors' official complaints are enormous, not only for the individual survivor but also for the whole constellation of family and friends. Indeed, when police statements were being drawn up while a survivor was still in therapy, they accounted for a significant part of the work we addressed. This related not only to the various practical issues involved, as well as the emotional and psychological effects on the survivor, but also as regards the post-complaint extensive interpersonal effects on the relationships between survivors and their families and partners. The topic merits extended discussion and this takes place in Chapter 12 about the families of survivors and also in Chapter 13 on recovered memory.

Drugs/alcohol/self-harm

Table 4.10 shows the frequency of women who reported difficulties in the areas of drugs, alcohol and self-harm. The table provides brief but relevant information on some variables that the women considered played an important part in the cluster of difficulties they presented with. When either one or a combination of these problems were reported, they frequently constituted the initial focus of intervention.

Table 4.10   Drugs, alcohol and self-harm

Category	Frequency	Percentage
Alcohol	13	7.2
Alcohol/drugs	4	2.2
Alcohol/self-harm	11	6.1
Drugs	2	1.1
Drugs/self-harm	2	1.1
Self-harm	19	10.6
Alcohol/drugs/self-harm	9	5.0
None	111	61.7
No data	9	5.0
Total	**180**	**100.0**

The overwhelming majority of survivors (61.7 per cent) said that they did not have problems with addiction of any sort and had never considered self-harm (i.e. self-mutilation and/or suicide attempts). There is no data for nine of the women, and of the rest of the sample of 180 women, 60 reported a problem with one or more of the categories. The most frequent problem reported (10.6 per cent) was self-harm, including self-mutilation and/or attempted suicide on one or more occasions. The second most problematic area was that of alcohol dependence and this accounted for 7 per cent of the women who volunteered such information. Nine of the women (5 per cent) admitted to problems in all areas and four women (2 per cent) reported problems with alcohol and drugs. Two women had problems with both drugs and self-harm and two with drugs only. When "drugs" are mentioned these refer to persistent and compulsive use ranging from cannabis smoking, Ecstasy, LSD, speed, heroin, and a variety of psychotropic drugs obtained on the black market. Occasional use of cannabis or other infrequent recreational use of drugs was not recorded, and neither were women on prescribed psychotropic medication (see the next sub-section).

Coping level

Table 4.11 provides a summary of the survivors' level of coping at initial presentation for psychological help. The distribution suggests that just over half of the women (52.7 per cent) appeared to cope with general aspects of life at varying degrees of satisfaction ranging from "OK" to "excellent". The rest (47.3 per cent) appeared to be having difficulty with coping, which ranged from "bad" to "very bad". Some explanation is required here about why the "coping" variable was included and also how it was measured.

Table 4.11   Coping level

Level	Frequency	Percentage
Very bad	30	16.7
Bad	55	30.6
OK	60	33.3
Quite well	33	18.3
Excellent	2	1.1
Total	**180**	**100.0**

The information was included because I considered that it was important for the reader to gain some appreciation, albeit very brief and general, about the manner in which survivors presented at their first session. While no assumptions are made here about long-term effects of sexual abuse, I wished to convey the women's subjective view of their ability to cope with certain aspects of life at the time of seeking help, combined with my own overall subjective interpretation of their level of coping. It is my opinion, based on clinical experience, that the issue of long-term effects following the experience of abuse is a very complex one. Indeed, I would go further to argue that the sheer complexity of the multifactorial nature of the relationship between personal and circumstantial variables renders the pursuit of "scientific accuracy" in this area at best reductionist and at worst lacking in accuracy. Nevertheless, for the benefit of readers not familiar with the literature on long-term effects, as well as for the sake of completeness, the next chapter addresses this issue.

Measurement of the degree of coping was based on a very simple "Global Rating". This is a one-sheet visual analogue scale adapted from Isaac Marks (1986) targeting the following areas: work; home management; social leisure activities; private leisure activities; and relationships/ communication with others (family, spouse, workmates, friends, etc.). This measure is routinely included in all adult patients' initial appointment letters, but there is no pressure or expectation that it will always be completed; it is sent in order to help patients identify the areas they wish to address. When the questionnaire was not completed, the areas in question were, nevertheless, addressed at the initial session. In this sense the measure is a subjective and arbitrary one, but I have found that it can be helpful in creating an initial focus. Indeed, survivors frequently express a desire to address immediate difficulties related to current experience, prior to embarking on the more difficult task of disclosure.

The five categories used to identify the level of coping, ranging from "excellent" to "very bad", were so graded according to my own subjective formulation as guided by the survivors' own subjective perception. Their verbal report, as well as their scores (when available) on an eight-point visual analogue scale ranging from "no problems at all" to "very severe problems", was used as a guide.

During the process of constructing my formulation of the extent of difficulties the women were expressing, many factors where reported by them as contributing to their distress and not all were attributed by them to the fact that they had been sexually abused. For example, women who perceived themselves as coping "very badly" would report problems with housing, difficult neighbours, stress in the workplace, financial difficulties, etc. This situation serves to underline my earlier comment with respect to the complexity of identifying the long-term effects of sexual abuse. In the next chapter dealing with this issue, more detailed examples will be discussed with reference to "level of coping", as summarised here.

Concluding issues

In ending this chapter I would like to summarise two other pertinent issues, in addition to those referred to above, brought to the consulting room by a number of women. The first refers to the very small number of women who requested therapy in order to address their concern about being abused in childhood by a "peer". This is an interesting issue and one that lacks clarity in terms of definition. The women in question expressed confusion as well as concern about the fact that although the perpetrator was, in all cases, not more than four years their senior, they nevertheless considered that they had been manipulated or coerced into participating in unwanted sexual activity. There does not seem to be consensus among professionals about when sexual activity amongst peers constitutes sexual abuse. So far, ages quoted have been arbitrary and they are usually qualified by adding that it is the maturity, power, and control of the initiator of sexual activity that defines this action as abusive. In the women I saw, there certainly appeared to be the perception that participation was unwanted and that there was a degree of coercion. It was also the case, however, in line with my arguments in the earlier section about media influence, that some women sought reassurance about a problem on which they were not altogether clear. In some cases, their verbal report indicated that there was a discrepancy between what they themselves believed had happened to them and what they perceived "others" to be saying. In the case of these few women whom I saw, brief counselling and/or reassurance appeared to be adequate intervention.

The second area I would like to refer to concerns another small group of women who sought help relating to feelings of concern and guilt about the fact that their children had been abused. I am certain that there must be numerous accounts of women presenting with these concerns, but I have found it interesting that in my case these particular women represent a very small proportion of the total number of women I have seen. I have come to realise that the role of mothers and their relationship to their daughters who have been abused is of crucial significance, and I discuss this issue in Chapter 13.

Long-term effects of sexual abuse: Empirical, theoretical, and clinical considerations

A GLOBAL PERSPECTIVE

In the first part of this chapter, I offer an overview of the literature that I have found to be relevant to my own work, while in the second part I discuss three theoretical models that attempt to conceptualise the long-term effects of childhood sexual abuse (CSA). In the final part of the chapter I focus on my own clinical experience with the survivors I have already introduced, with particular reference to their subjective reports relating to the aftermath of their abuse. Here, special attention will be given to survivors' differing levels of self-efficacy or "coping", and it is hoped that the discussion of subjective as well as clinical observations will impart a body of information that might be helpful to other practitioners.

A review of the CSA literature reflects a mixed if not confusing picture. Although there has been a steady increase in journal publications concerned with the issue of CSA since the middle of the 1980s, few studies of the sequelae of CSA have been undertaken. Moreover, as with publications on the prevalence of CSA, those concerned with its long-term effects suffer with the same methodological problems, such as self-selected samples; lack of appropriate controls; small or "captive" populations; the use of arbitrary, non-inclusive, and differential variables; inadequate statistical analyses; and, of course, differential definitions of what is meant by sexual abuse. Moreover, while the degree of negative impact following CSA varies considerably (Coffey et al, 1996), Fleming et al (1999) suggests that, ". . . the issue of the exact role of CSA in the etiology of adverse negative outcomes will remain highly controversial and contentious". The writer asserts, however, that this should not thwart our commitment in this very important area of investigation.

Indeed, despite these difficulties, we should feel indebted to those who have heralded the wave of growing interest in the field of CSA in general, and its long-term effects in particular. Finkelhor (1979, 1980, 1984, 1988, 1990, 1991) has been an important contributor and his update of long-term effects (Finkelhor, 1990) lists CSA sequelae such as low self-esteem, reduced self-efficacy, depression, anxiety, and sexual/interpersonal problems. Such findings fit in with subsequent reviews on long-term effects (Cahil et al, 1991; Beitchman et al, 1992). However, more recent publications have begun to unravel a more complex picture, and although there is no argument about the fact that the sequelae mentioned above are indeed evident in many adult survivors of CSA, they only relate to a small part of this much wider and multifaceted picture.

Although low self-esteem, for example, has been found to be an important long-term effect in a number of studies (Gold, 1986; Bagley and Ramsay, 1986; Hart et al, 1989; Lundberg-Love, 1990; Romans et al, 1996; Fleming et al, 1999), including those based on the experience of clinicians (Courtois, 1988; Jehu, 1988; Sanderson, 1990; Kirschner et al, 1993; Kennerley, 2000) and survivors alike, it has not been looked at in relation to its adjuncts—i.e. self-confidence, self-efficacy, and perceived competence. I would contend that self-esteem and self-confidence, for example, are two separate entities, where the first is the private measure of an individual's personal worth and the second represents the varying degrees to which this measure is made evident to others. Each of the many survivors of CSA whom I have seen, presents with their own particular measure of self-worth, with equal individuality about the degree to which this translates to self-confidence, belief in competencies, and general self-efficacy. It is not unusual, for example, for a survivor to comment that although she feels like "rubbish inside" when she is socialising, she is perfectly competent in her work and even "fools" people with her projection of efficacy. It would be crucial, therefore, that when lowered self-esteem is discussed as being an important sequel to CSA, that self-efficacy as well as self-confidence are examined, with particular attention to the factors that lead to survivors' individual perceptions and presentations. Indeed, while "lowered self-efficacy" has been described as being another important sequel of CSA, this has not been empirically studied in conjunction with self-esteem, or in terms of the many different areas in which efficacy might be measured.

In some psychological studies, attention has been given to survivors' negative self-attributions. Such work has made a very useful contribution in the treatment of adult survivors because it attempts to "unpack" some of the issues I raised in the previous paragraph. In particular, the work of Jehu et al (1985/6) and Jehu (1988) demonstrated the effectiveness of cognitive restructuring in reducing symptoms of mood disturbance in adult CSA survivors, while a study by Wenninger and Ehlers (1998) suggested a relationship between inflexible attributional style and post-traumatic symptoms. Although these contributions have gone some way towards attending to CSA survivors' individual belief systems about themselves and the impact these might have on their mood and clinical presentation, there continues to be a lack of attention to the competencies that many survivors have irrespective of their belief system.

The next long-term effect in adult survivors of CSA which has received much attention is depression. Following the early work of Finkelhor, corroboration of its importance was found in a number of subsequent investigations (Mullen et al, 1988; Pribor and Dinwiddie, 1992; Mullen et al, 1993; Yama et al, 1993; Bifulco and Moran, 1998; Weiss et al, 1999). Weiss et al (1999), however, rightfully point out that other types of childhood trauma (concurrently or otherwise)—such as parental loss, domestic violence and/or alcoholism, parental mental illness, as well as poor parenting—could all have a bearing on vulnerability to depression. Moreover, a more recent study (Melchert, 2000), which attempted to clarify the effects of CSA, parental substance abuse, and parental caregiving on adult adjustment, concluded that an absence of respectful approval, particularly from the mother, was at least as important as parental substance abuse and CSA in predicating adult psychological distress.

These very pertinent conclusions highlight the fact that while we should be vigilant as clinicians in monitoring the presence of clinical depression in survivors of CSA, we should be equally aware that not all survivors become depressed and, most importantly, that other factors apart from the abuse itself might be more relevant to those who are depressed. To date, I have not reviewed a paper that has successfully combined and then differentiated between these other childhood traumas when assessing the incidence of depression in CSA survivors—particularly in those who, in addition to CSA, have also experienced one or more of the above traumas. As I mentioned at the start of this chapter, however, the more recent studies are beginning to acknowledge the complexity of attributing long-term effects to any one variable in the experience of CSA survivors. Indeed, the timely acknowledgement that the family of origin might be, if not more important than the abuse itself, at least as important in determining a survivor's later life adjustment, can be found in a number of publications.

A review of the empirical literature on the long-term correlates of CSA by Polusny and Follette (1995) concluded that while there were mixed findings for an association between CSA and social isolation and social adjustment, there was a suggestion in the available data that both sexual abuse and family of origin characteristics were relevant variables for further research. Indeed, that the atmosphere in the family of origin substantially accounts for the variance of all measures of psychopathology has been corroborated in a number of studies (Nash et al, 1993; Yama et al, 1993; Faust et al, 1995; Spacarelli and Fuchs, 1997). Moreover, a more recent study by Lange et al (1999) which subjected the above results to univariate analyses suggested not only that the latter's findings held for both incestuous and non-incestuous abuse, but in addition found confirmation in their own sample of 404 women that the emotional atmosphere in the family of origin, reactions after disclosure, and self-blame, were more strongly associated with later psychopathology than objective characteristics of the abuse itself. Certainly, in my own work with female survivors of CSA, the issue of self-blame, lack of parental validation of the abuse, and a generally non-supportive and unprotective family environment have all been offered, in varying degrees, by them as being the major contributors to their current distress.

Complexities and contradictions

The literature on the relationship between sexual abuse characteristics and long-term effects is inconclusive, particularly in the light of the above discussion. Although variables such as nature of perpetrator, type of abuse, duration and frequency of abuse, and age at the onset of abuse have received much attention, there is a lack of consensus about their specific long-term effects. For example, multivariate analyses by Binder et al (1996) to identify variables that predicted psychological well-being of adult female survivors of CSA concluded that short duration of abuse, absence of perceived pressure, and absence of family conflict emerged as important predictors of well-being, in spite of type of abuse. On the other hand, Briggs and Joyce (1997), who sought to determine which CSA characteristics were related to post-traumatic symptomatology, concluded that having multiple abusive episodes that involved intercourse significantly predicted scores on hyperarousal, intrusive thoughts, and dissociation. The study did not, however, control for the relationship between perpetrator and survivor and other family dynamics.

More recently, in a study by Fleming et al (1999), which targeted a randomly selected sample of 6,000 Australian women and sought to evaluate the long-term impact of CSA, it was concluded that those women who had been exposed to CSA involving penetration were at greater risk of later victimisation, such as rape and domestic violence. The same study also confirmed that a history of CSA, in general was associated with poor quality of women's relationships in adult life, and that they were likely to report that their partners were highly controlling.

The above are only a few examples of the contradictions that beset the literature on specific abuse characteristics and their long-term effects. In my decade's work as clinician with large numbers of CSA survivors, the published work that I have found to be of most relevance and help when attempting to conceptualise their experience and its effects is that which emphasises the importance of family dynamics (as discussed earlier); this issue is examined further in Chapter 13, and its impact is also apparent in the individual case studies.

Equally relevant have been the issues of "coping" and perceived self-blame or responsibility for the abuse. Morrow and Sorell (1989), in particular, highlighted the importance of subjective factors and coping behaviour, and demonstrated that survivors who held the perpetrator responsible for their abuse reported fewer psychiatric symptoms when compared with those who attributed responsibility to themselves. Although some subsequent studies have looked at these issues (e.g. Mennen and Meadow, 1994), there continues to be a dearth of surveys that focus on eliciting the subjective coping strategies of both "well" and "unwell" survivors of CSA. Such work could provide invaluable insights for our understanding of how survivors construe their abuse and which individual factors determine their personal adaptation or lack of it.

I hope that I have, so far, managed to illustrate some of the complexities involved in our understanding of the sequelae of CSA, and I am aware that I have yet to address a host of other long-term difficulties that have received attention. Eating disorders, sexual problems, anxiety, social functioning, drug and alcohol dependence, revictimisation, and self-harm have all been mentioned in the literature, both empirical and clinical, but without sufficient consensus, clarity, or distinction. There has existed, for some time, the belief that the experience of sexual abuse is linked with eating disorders (Oppenheimer et al, 1985; Root and Fallon, 1988; Courtois, 1988; Andrews, Valentine, and Valentine, 1995). Although clinically this can be said to be the case, the agreement is no more than a generalised observation from the tip of a vast iceberg. Here are some observations. First, it would be true to say that the idea of shape, size, and weight appears to be an endemic preoccupation for most women in the Western world (Grogan, 2000). There are, of course, degrees of concern ranging from mild awareness that one may wish to look more desirable, according to which trend prevails at any particular time, to maladaptive and destructive obsession about weight. In this sense, an "eating concern" might be argued to be a continuum along which any woman might lie at any one time, and this includes survivors of CSA.

Secondly, my own observation of the survivors I have worked with is that they generally fall into three groups with respect to body image and weight. The first group, which ranks second largest of the three, is made up of survivors who do not appear to have significantly greater concerns than the general population of women I have seen to date. The second, and smallest group, is made up of those survivors who present with distinct eating disorders, such as anorexia, bulimia, and obesity. Indeed, in my clinical experience this group is actually smaller than that of women with such disorders whom I have seen in the absence of CSA. The third and largest group has been that of survivors who reported a negative body image in general and for whom "dysfunctional eating" has been a means of manipulating and controlling the source of their distress as distinct from wishing to be thinner per se. Moreover, there is no observable consistency or method to their maladaptive eating. What makes this particular group different from women who have similar body dysphoria is that the survivors of CSA tend to attribute the distaste towards their bodies to the sexual abuse they have experienced, and view it as the source of their discontent.

The third important observation, and one that has recently received attention (Kent et al, 1999), is that emotional abuse may be even more important in the development of eating disorders than sexual abuse. Once more, therefore, the need for distinction between important variables is highlighted when studying the long-term effects of CSA, and the context for such study needs to be significantly widened.

The issue of "sexual problems" is a further contentious area. As a general rule there is a belief that because the nature of the abuse was sexual, many survivors of CSA will experience difficulties in their adult sexual relationships. Once again, however, there has been a tendency towards generalisation based on small or clinical samples and, in my opinion, more specificity is required. More crucially, DiLillo and Long (1999) argue that although numerous clinical texts have highlighted the relationship between detrimental effects of couple functioning and the experience of CSA (Malz, 1988; Kristberg, 1990; Davis, 1991; Engle, 1991; Gil, 1992; Stark, 1993), only a few empirical studies (e.g. Finkelhor et al, 1989; Mullen et al, 1994) have looked at the specific relationship characteristics of the survivor.

In my own clinical experience with survivors of CSA, I have found the picture relating to sexual difficulties to be less than straightforward. Indeed, my interest in women who had experienced sexual abuse in their childhood developed at the start of my career as a clinical psychologist, and more specifically, in my role of psychosexual therapist. I became aware that women referred from a number of agencies (mostly medical as opposed to psychiatric) over a three-year period for sexual difficulties (Baker, 1992) would frequently relate an experience of CSA. The most common complaint among these women was a lack of interest in sex and/or dissatisfaction with their sexual relationships in general, rather than a specific dysfunction such as anorgasmia, vaginismus, or dyspareunia. Moreover, as regards joint sessions with partners, it was evident that straightforward contractual interventions requiring the collaboration of the couple to carry out "task assignments" between sessions would not be appropriate.

During the course of my work over a decade ago with couples where the female partner was a survivor of CSA, I gained a great deal of insight into the complexity of the survivors' sexuality and their personal conflicts. These encompassed a whole host of issues, in particular inability to trust; powerlessness; negative body image; dissociation; flashbacks of the abuse during certain intimate moments; negative feelings about sex; inability to relax; insecurity and morbid jealousy; controlling behaviour; and poor communication skills. It was my observation of these issues, as well as their manifestation in differing combinations and degrees of severity, which led to a growing interest in working on an individual basis with female survivors of CSA. I became aware that "sexual difficulties" in the clinical context was at best a generic term that encompassed a survivor's inability to negotiate a satisfying and stable emotional relationship, and within which the sexual dimension was subjectively perceived as having a controlling role.

A further and very pertinent observation was that most survivors were indeed able, under certain conditions, to enjoy sex and even actively seek it. The latter appeared to be particularly the case at the start of a new relationship, followed by a gradual decline in sexual activity once the relationship had been established, and particularly after the couple had been cohabiting for some time. In-depth exploration of this observation helped to unravel the complexity of the issues I mentioned earlier. For example, the women frequently related that in the early stages of a new relationship, where there was perceived potential for a future, a great emotional investment appeared to override any anxieties related to their previous abuse. It was only once the relationship was established and couple intimacy, on many levels, became the norm within the context of cohabitation, that the problems began. Indeed, I was to discover that for the most severely affected survivors the nightmare of their CSA was to start unravelling once they were well engaged in a long-term relationship, and particularly after their own children were born. These issues are discussed further in subsequent chapters of the book, and will be made more explicit in the detailed presentation of case studies. Suffice to say at this stage, that any study of sexual difficulties in adult survivors of CSA must take into account emotional, perceptual, and couple functioning variables.

Moreover, attention needs to be paid to the male partners of survivors in terms of their own coping resources and attitudes to their partners' abuse. Currently, there is a dearth of work on this issue, which, in my opinion, requires urgent attention if we are to effectively help couples with a history of CSA. In my own clinical practice I was hugely helped by reading the paper on partners of female survivors of CSA by Firth (1997). In it he succinctly outlines potential difficulties for these partners, such as *fear* of discovering their own potential for CSA (or—my addition—their own past abuse); *anger* towards the abuser, the survivor, and themselves; *guilt and/or shame* about their own sexual impulses, leading to *inhibition and lack of spontaneity*; and *disempowerement* through their partners' need to be completely in control of all aspects of their relationship. These issues can be focal points within the joint therapeutic context, which in many instances is a vital adjunct to the individual sessions with female survivors.

Of course not all survivors who present for therapy are in stable relationships, and very frequently their complaint is that they are unable to sustain them, while other survivors actively avoid them. These, as well as other long-term effects that have not yet been discussed—such as promiscuity, revictimisation, alcohol and drug abuse, and self-harm—are subsumed, along with "relationship difficulties", in the discussion that follows of three models which attempt to conceptualise the long-term effects of CSA.

THEORETICAL MODELS

Having already raised the difficulties involved in establishing a relationship between specific long-term effects of CSA and any of the multitude of variables that were highlighted earlier, the issue of mediational factors (i.e. between the experience of CSA and problems with later adjustment) remains largely unexplained. Although cognitive factors are relevant in understanding survivors' perceptions, we are still unclear about how these perceptions are actually mediated. Clearly a host of both internal as well as external influences could be involved, such as the child's personal resources and degree of self-sufficiency; circumstances of the disclosure or lack of it; other people's reactions to survivors and sexual abuse in general; and the level of parental validation and support.

Coffey et al (1996) point out that in order to determine, for example, whether particular feelings such as stigma or self-blame developmentally influence adjustment or whether adjustment influences feelings of stigma and self-blame, the methodological design most likely to provide these answers would have to be a prospective one that begins in childhood when the abuse first occurred. The authors correctly point out, however, that only a minority of survivors report their abuse during childhood (which has certainly been the case in my own clinical experience). Nevertheless, in spite of the difficulties inherent in our search for an accurate understanding of how long-term effects of CSA are mediated, a number of theoretical models have been proposed that can help, if only partly, towards a conceptualisation of survivors' difficulties. In the remainder of this section, I discuss those found to be particularly helpful when treating survivors of sexual abuse.

Traumagenic dynamics

This model was proposed in 1985 by Finkelhor and Browne. It attempts to explain a broad range of CSA sequelae and posits that sexual abuse negatively affects a child's cognitive and affective orientations to the world, resulting in disturbances in four domains or "dynamics": *betrayal; powerlessness; stigmatisation; and traumatic sexualisation.* Table 5.1 summarises the psychological and behavioural implications in each of these dynamics.

The traumagenic model has been a very helpful guide, particularly in the early days of my work in the CSA area, in that it highlights four important domains that incorporate a number of pertinent difficulties that survivors present with. However, the model has its limitations:

1. Although it offers insights for clinical conceptualisation, none of the posited dynamics has been conclusively established through empirical study as having a relationship to adult adjustment.

Table 5.1   The traumagenic model (based on the work of Finkelhor and Browne, 1985 and 1986)

Dynamics	Psychological impacts	Behavioural sequelae
Betrayal Violation of expectation of care and protection from others; there is no support and protection from parents; trust and vulnerability are manipulated.	Depression; mistrust and impaired ability to judge trustworthiness; anger; dependency.	Delinquency; isolation; re-victimisation; insecurity; marital/relationship problems; inadequate parenting; aggression.
Powerlessness Coercion (psychological or physical) is used to involve children; body territory is invaded against the child's wishes; inability to make others believe disclosures; living with perpetual fear and vulnerability; and (my addition) the adults' needs are superior to the child's.	Poor self-efficacy and perception of self as victim; fear and anxiety; identification with the perpetrator; depression; nightmares; phobias.	Need to control; eating disorders; truancy; dissociation; bullying; becoming a perpetrator; and (my additions) subjugation of personal needs; lack of assertiveness; poor personal boundaries; learned helplessness.
Stigmatisation Others behave in any one (or combination) of the following ways: pressure children for secrecy; blame children for the abuse and/or react negatively to disclosure; perpetrators humiliate and blame the victims for the abuse.	Internalisation of feelings of guilt and shame about the abuse; feeling different from other people; low self-worth; and (my additions) perceived defectiveness; social anxiety and undesirability.	Social isolation and avoidance; alcohol and substance abuse; self-harm; suicide attempts; and (my addition) poor social integration.
Traumatic sexualisation Perpetrators engage in the following: they "groom" children through the use of attention and affection in order to gratify their sexual needs; they fetishise sexual parts of children; they convey a distorted picture of sexual morality; they reward their victims for sexual acts that are inappropriate to their developmental level.	Sexual activity is associated with negative memories and emotions; confusion about the role of sex in loving and caring relationships; disrupted sexual identity; confusion about sexual norms; aversion to sex; fear of intimacy.	Premature sexualisation and preoccupation with sex; compulsive sexual behaviours; avoidance of sex and/or phobias about specific acts; promiscuity; prostitution; impaired arousal; flashbacks; and either inappropriate sexualisation of parenting, or (my additions) excessive preoccupation with safety of children; fear of becoming a perpetrator.

2. Not all survivors have difficulties in all four dynamics and there is great survivor variation in terms of which dynamics are an issue in adult life.
3. Finkelhor and Browne (1985) described the traumagenic dynamics at the time of the abuse during childhood, but the factors that mediate the development of each dynamic have not been addressed.

Very little work has been undertaken to address some of these issues. The most recent comprehensive study I have been able to find is that of Coffey et al (1996). The writers used a community sample of 192 adult women who had experienced CSA and attempted to test the hypothesis that betrayal, powerlessness, perceived stigma, and self-blame mediated the long-term effects of CSA. Using path analysis, they found partial support for the traumagenic dynamics model suggesting that stigma and self-blame acted as mediators for the current psychological distress experienced by the survivors of CSA. Certainly, in my experience, the women who expressed the most self-blame were those who felt the most defective and who had great difficulty recognising and addressing their individual needs. These, as well as other issues raised by the traumagenic model will be discussed further in the "Observations" section later in this chapter, in terms of implications for personal development and level of coping. In Chapter 13, family variables that could act as possible mediators for feelings of stigmatisation and self-blame will also be addressed.

Post-traumatic stress disorder

Post-traumatic stress disorder (PTSD) is a recognised syndrome associated with having experienced an event outside the range of normally expected human experience (DSM-IV, American Psychiatric Association, 1994). Documented examples of such events include, but are not limited to military combat, road traffic accidents, natural disasters, torture, incarceration as a prisoner of war or in a concentration camp, and experiencing violent personal assault (e.g. physical attack, mugging, and sexual assault). The requirements for a diagnosis of PTSD are that symptoms in each of the following categories are experienced for at least one month or longer:

1. The event is persistently re-experienced through distressing dreams, flashbacks, and recurrent intrusive recollections of the event.
2. The person engages in persistent avoidance of stimuli associated with the trauma—e.g. thoughts and feelings associated with the traumatic event, inability to recall an important aspect of the trauma, situations or activities that trigger recollections of the trauma.
3. Persistent symptoms of arousal, especially sleep-related problems, hypervigilance, irritability, and startled response.

The attempt to conceptualise the long-term difficulties of survivors of CSA within a model of PTSD is relatively recent. Some authors contend that symptoms of PTSD are almost universal in adult survivors of CSA (e.g. Lindberg and Distad, 1985; Goodwin, 1990; Herman, 1992), while others have concluded that only a minority of survivors are troubled by the syndrome (e.g. McLeer et al, 1988; Resnick et al, 1993). More recently, Briggs and Joyce (1997), in a study of seventy-three women attending a Family Health Counselling Service's Sexual Abuse Programme in New Zealand, concluded that the severity of PTSD symptoms was associated with the extent to which CSA involved sexual intercourse. The authors also suggested that many women who experienced CSA endorsed symptoms of PTSD, and that the severity of the latter correlated with the extent of general psychopathology. It is unclear, however, what is meant by "many women", or what types of specific psychopathology are being referred to.

In a study of female primary care patients with a history of CSA, Dickinson et al (1998) found support for the existence of a complex PTSD syndrome, but only in one of four identified clusters of survivors. Of the ninety-nine women who took part in the study, thirty-five (cluster 1) presented with least symptomatology. The survivors in this group tended to have experienced less severe abuse, less incestuous abuse, and little domestic violence. Survivors in clusters 2, 3, and 4 showed high levels of depressive and somatic symptoms, and all had experienced more severe CSA than the women in cluster 1; in addition, there was no difference between them with respect to prevalence of incest, severity, or duration of abuse. However, there were differences among them with respect to rates of domestic violence, physical abuse, and combined abuse. The authors concluded that severe and prolonged abuse, particularly if this was in conjunction with violence and a generally chaotic family environment, was associated with greater symptomatology and dissociative symptoms. Interestingly, however, only 30 per cent of the overall sample qualified for a diagnosis of PTSD; these were the survivors relegated to cluster 4. Here, the women had histories of severe sexual abuse, frequently combined with physical abuse, criminal and violent behaviour in the family environment, and multiple forms of abuse. The presenting symptomatology included depression, PTSD symptoms, dissociative symptoms, alcohol abuse, and somatic complaints.

Further research in this area is much needed because the existing work that attempts to describe survivors' symptoms in terms of a PTSD syndrome is rather sparse and involves small clinical samples. In my own work I have found the number of survivors who present with a frank PTSD syndrome to be relatively small. However, this is particularly the case when one adheres to the standard DSM-IV classification (American Psychiatric Association, 1994). A further group of survivors whom I have seen also present with particular aspects of PTSD—namely intrusive thoughts, avoidance of certain sexual behaviours, and disturbed sleep with nightmares—but they do not comply with the DSM-IV criteria. The remaining group of female survivors (approximately 40 per cent) whom I presented in Chapter 4 reported no post-traumatic symptoms as defined in the PTSD literature. Clearly, more empirical work is required that could help towards a more comprehensive assessment of survivors' presenting complaints, as well as more effective and prompt intervention when necessary.

In spite of the limitations of the PTSD model in relation to CSA, I have personally found it to be of particular relevance and help when assessing the complaints of the more distressed survivors. The main benefits have been two-fold. First, it has contributed towards the accuracy and completion of my formulation within (usually) very complex sets of presenting problems. Secondly, it has enabled me to take prompt and specific therapeutic action by requesting pharmacological referral, and/or through the adoption of specific therapeutic techniques when appropriate, such as imagery, exposure, and desensitisation. Indeed, as will be made more explicit later in this book, imagery with rescripting is particularly (and possibly only) appropriate and most effective when a survivor presents with severe PTSD symptoms (Smucker et al, 1995).

In my own clinical experience, the presence of frank PTSD has been infrequent, and most likely to be one of several other difficulties a survivor is having to negotiate. Moreover, it has been most evident among the group of survivors who belong to the category of coping "badly" or "very badly" (see Chapter 4). There is further discussion on this issue in the final section of this chapter.

Borderline personality disorder

The last model I would like to discuss here in relation to conceptualising the long-term effects on survivors of CSA is that of borderline personality disorder. It must be made clear from the outset that as a broad principle, not only in my treatment of survivors of CSA but also in other adults in general, I prefer conceptualisations that do not automatically or unnecessarily pathologise the clients. This approach is born out of a belief that mental distress is a continuum along which anyone can lie at a particular time in their life. This is, of course, a very general perspective but nevertheless one that allows me to maximise a client's existing competencies in preference to marginalising specific psychological complaints and labelling them as psychiatric or pathological. However, any responsible clinician would seek to eliminate or target Axis I disorder (i.e. clinical syndromes that require immediate intervention—either psychological and/or pharmacological—such as major depression, PTSD, and eating disorders). Equally, I have been made aware that I would not be carrying out my duty as a clinician if I were to ignore pervasive patterns of behaviour that repeatedly lead to intense distress and that can frequently be accompanied by self-destructive behaviour. The more I have undertaken in-depth work with clients—i.e. survivors of childhood abuse in general, and CSA in particular—the more I have appreciated the importance of remaining vigilant to Axis II features, namely borderline personality disorder (American Psychiatric Association, 1994). This became especially the case when it was evident that problem-solving cognitive/behavioural techniques alone were either inadequate or even threatening to some survivors, particularly in the first stages of their therapy (see Zanarini, 1997; Linehan, 1998).

Chapters 6, 7, and 8 include extensive discussion of the issues I have raised, and they are examined in terms of the role of the therapist, theoretical integration, survivors' need for validation, and clinical intervention. The remainder of this section provides an overview of the literature on borderline personality disorder (BPD), an area in which there has been little empirical research in terms of its specific relationship to CSA. One of the most documented aspects of BPD in relation to CSA is the demonstration that overall rates of CSA (i.e. incestuous and non-incestuous) reported by borderline patients range from 16 per cent to 71 per cent (Herman et al, 1989; Ogata et al, 1990; Western et al, 1990; Salzman et al, 1993; Zanarini et al, 1997), whilst in up to 30 per cent, the CSA reported involved a full-time adult care taker (Zanarini et al, 1989; Links et al, 1988; Ogata et al, 1990; Western et al, 1990; Shearer et al, 1993). In the study by Zanarini et al (1997), the general conclusion was that CSA was neither sufficient nor necessary for the development of BPD. However, some further important issues were suggested: first, for about half of their sample (115 male and female in-patients), CSA appeared to be an important etiological factor for BPD; secondly, this abuse occurred mostly within a chaotic family atmosphere and biparental neglect; and thirdly, in the other half of the patients other types of abuse (i.e. emotional, physical, verbal), in conjunction with neglect, was argued to play a more central etiological role. These conclusions provide important insights, particularly for clinicians. Indeed, my own perception of survivors of sexual abuse has been that the most severely affected survivors (i.e. whose current distress conforms to the criteria for BPD) tend to express at least an equal, and often more severe distress, to other childhood experiences that were neglectful and/or abusive. Along these lines, Zanarini et al (1997) conclude their study by highlighting the most striking characteristic of BPD as being the enormous inner pain that is experienced, and emphasise the patients' need for validation before they begin their journey to health. This very pertinent observation will be illustrated in the case studies in Chapters 9, 10, and 11.

Although the work on BPD in relation to CSA is still in its infancy, a number of other related issues have received attention. One of these is the relationship of CSA to dissociation and self-mutilation in female patients. Dissociation is conceptualised as "a pathological failure to integrate thoughts, feelings, and memories into a coherent, unified sense of consciousness" (Brodsky et al, 1995, p. 1788). Zweig-Frank and Paris (1997), to their surprise, found that although dissociation was indeed higher in a sample of female patients with BPD, these scores bore no significant relationship to CSA per se, even though incestuous as well as non-incestuous abuse was included. Their findings are in direct contrast with other studies that had found an association between CSA and dissociation (Chu and Dill, 1990; Kirby et al, 1993; Ogata et al, 1990). Zweig-Frank and Paris (1997) explain this contrast in terms of the following factors: the first two studies employed no diagnosis at all, while the third had not separated the diagnosis of BPD from the specific abuse history in relation to dissociation. Moreover, Zweig-Frank and Paris (1997) support the validity of their findings by pointing out the fact that the size of their sample was larger than that of any previous report, and that their results replicated those of a previous study that had utilised an equally large sample of men.

Clearly, more research is needed in this area, particularly because there has been a tendency, mainly by clinicians, to link the experience of CSA with dissociation. Moreover, there could be huge implications regarding the continuing contentious debate about the validity of survivors' recollections of their abuse. The issue of false/recovered memories will be discussed further in Chapter 14, but I would like to offer my own observations about dissociation, which is one of the many facets of CSA that I have found to be inconsistent. Certainly, it has not been a feature that I have observed only in survivors of CSA, or indeed in all of them. The inability to make connections in one's behaviour over time, and the repetition of inappropriate choices and destructive behaviours without apparent insight, are issues that I have addressed in patients with BPD, irrespective of CSA. The strongest link between all of these patients has been their perception of a deeply unhappy childhood, with or without sexual abuse.

Emotional neglect and the lack of attendance to a survivor's individual personality and needs during their childhood, or as many patients plainly put it, "I was not heard, and often wondered if I belonged to my family", appeared to have had a significant impact on them. It is therefore possible that it is the cumulative effect of many types of abuse and neglect towards a child that can mediate the development of BPD, and dissociation in particular. Indeed, dissociation, especially when the experience of abuse in childhood is severe, is argued to be an adaptive response to an environment that is perceived as cruel, frightening, inconsistent, punishing, degrading, invalidating, and neglecting of the child. It is in adolescence and adulthood that dissociation may account for the pervasive patterns of maladaptive and destructive behaviour. The point is once more emphasised that the clinician's primary role is to validate the client's experience if any trust is to be built (see Chapter 7).

A biosocial perspective has also been proposed in explaining the development of destructive behaviour and its relationship to CSA; this will be looked at a little later in this section, but I would first like to complete the discussion about dissociation in relation to self-mutilation. The study by Zweig-Frank and Paris (1997) suggested, as in the case of dissociation, that although CSA discriminated borderline from non-borderline personality disorders, it did not discriminate between BPD patients who self-mutilated and those who did not. Moreover, none of the CSA parameters, including penetration, nor levels of dissociation were significant discriminating factors. In view of their negative results, the authors attempt to explain them in terms of two propositions. First, that self-mutilation might be accounted for, at least in part, by biological factors (e.g. trait impulsivity) and quote some empirical evidence for a relationship between impulsive aggression and reduced serotonergic activity (Coccaro et al, 1989; Markowitz, 1993). Secondly, they refer to the notion of "social contagion" (Walsh and Rosen, 1985) and suggest that patients with BPD perhaps begin their self-harming behaviour by imitation and not as a result of childhood experiences.[1]

I consider the last two statements to be very general observations and certainly not reflective of the histories recounted by survivors of CSA. Although they might contain some truth, they are missing important points about the emotional pain that I have repeatedly encountered in my clinical practice. I found the conclusions of Dudo et al (1997) based on a study that looked at the relationship between "lifetime self-destructiveness and patho-logical childhood experiences", to be much more insightful and relevant to clinical practice. First, the authors identified a subgroup of survivors (5 per cent of a sample of forty-two women who met the criteria for BPD) who began to self-mutilate in early childhood, while 12 per cent had made suicide attempts between the ages of six and twelve. Secondly, the authors conclude that both CSA and neglect by a caregiver play an important role in the etiology of self-harm (this includes both self-mutilation and suicide attempts). Moreover, when the abuse occurred in a generally non-protective and invali-dating environment, the neglectful features of the patients' family environ-ment gained etiological importance. Finally, and most importantly, Dudo et al (1997) acknowledge that the study of self-harm requires the adoption of a multifactorial perspective and also that attempts to conceptualise it might be carried out in terms of different theories—e.g. psychodynamic, develop-mental (see Chapter 13), and biological. In addition, they point out the communicative role of self-destructive behaviour in patients with BPD, in their desperate attempt to convey their anger, pain, and disappointment towards their families and also the professionals who attempt to help them. This will be clearly illustrated in two of the case studies (Chapters 10 and 11).

Biosocial aspects of CSA

I will conclude this section with a discussion of Wagner and Linehan's (1997) biosocial perspective on the relationship between CSA and BPD, and the role of suicidal behaviour. The authors begin by affirming the strong association between CSA and the diagnosis of BPD, but do not assert that sexual abuse causes BPD. Indeed, they point out that not all people with BPD report histories of sexual abuse, and also that many people who report such histories do not develop BPD. Their proposed explanation for these variations is illustrated using a "biosocial theory" of BPD which argues that a fundamental disruption of an individual's emotion regulation system arises from a combination of "biological vulnerability" to emotions and an "invalidating environment". The biological components are speculated to be a combination of genetic influences (e.g. affective disorder, alcoholism, and drug abuse in first degree relatives), harmful intrauterine events (e.g. malnutrition, environmental stress, substance abuse), and developmental factors (e.g. neurological development and childhood trauma) that can "dysregulate" physiological and emotional development. Although Wagner and Linehan (1997) do point out that there is currently insufficient empirical support for the relationship between biological vulnerability and development of BPD, they nevertheless contend that such vulnerability can have an impact on information-processing via the limbic system, which is the primary neurological system for the integration of incoming information (see Hartman and Burgess, 1993). Indeed, it is hypothesised that childhood trauma and CSA, in particular, might actually overwhelm the limbic system to such a degree that it could precipitate heightened emotional arousal and emotion dysregulation in response to events or situations, thus causing biological vulnerability in abused children by permanently altering their central nervous system.

An invalidating environment is one that does not take into account vulnerability as discussed above. Hence, not all children who are born with emotional vulnerability or who have experienced sexual abuse go on to develop BPD. According to the biosocial theory (Wagner and Linehan, 1997), children who are most likely to develop BPD are those whose vulnerability is disrespected, ignored, and invalidated. For example, emotional and cognitive reactions or behaviours in a child are persistently treated as being invalid responses to events (see Linehan, 1993) or are met with inconsistent, punishing, and other extreme emotional reactions. According to the authors, CSA represents the ultimate invalidation due to three factors previously identified by Finkelhor and Browne (1986):

1. Invasion of the child's body.
2. Confusion about the meaning of the abuse. For example, society or the family might express condemnation about CSA, while the child is being abused by a family member.
3. Breach of trust; the child is either let down in his/her expectation of safety in the family environment, or is not protected by the family when the perpetrator is outside it.

Other invalidating aspects include the issue of secrecy and inappropriate responses by the family when disclosure occurs (Courtois, 1988). When a child is asked to keep the abuse secret, he/she is not allowed to seek external validation for their internal feelings and reactions. This creates dependency on the perpetrator who has to be relied on to provide meaning to the child's experience. If or when the abuse is disclosed, the typically invalidating environment will deny, rationalise, or minimise the abuse, especially if it is incestuous. Indeed, the child might actually be blamed for the abuse.

Given these crucial issues, Wagner and Linehan (1997) assert that, for survivors of CSA who have BPD, the validation of their experience is of particular importance. This latter assertion is one that I unequivocally believe in, whether survivors have BPD or not. This issue is discussed in depth in Chapters 6 and 7, and illustrated in the extended case studies that follow.

The biosocial perspective offers, in addition, important insights about the role of suicidal behaviour in clients with BPD, and, in particular, those who have histories of CSA (Landecker, 1992). Wagner and Linehan (1997) argue that suicide ideation, suicide threats, and parasuicidal acts are not only common in individuals diagnosed with BPD, but that these acts discriminate BPD from all other personality disorders (e.g. Zanarini et al, 1990). The authors propose two main functions of suicidal behaviour: emotion regulation and a means of getting help. In the first instance, following parasuicidal acts, survivors explain their behaviour as an attempt to escape their feelings of anger, pain, shame, and anxiety. In the second instance, a survivor's perception that only extreme measures are likely to receive attention might reinforce suicidal behaviour, because it is seen as the most effective means of influencing a generally invalidating environment. Further reinforcement might, in addition, be unwittingly conveyed by therapists or medical professionals if they respond with concern and immediacy only when extreme measures are taken by the patient. I tend to agree with these propositions concerning suicidal behaviour, and I am particularly aware of the manipulative power that this can have on professionals. These issues are clearly demonstrated in Chapter 11, especially in terms of their importance within a framework of BPD.

In closing this discussion on BPD, I wish to convey that I have found it to be quite a significant factor in those survivors who have presented with the most severe long-term effects of their experience of childhood abuse in general, and sexual abuse in particular. Indeed, by paying attention to this diagnosis in the context of my own conceptualisation of their difficulties, I have been able to be vigilant to their emotional pain and despair, and to continually reappraise my own behaviour, as well as therapeutic stance and practice. I would go as far as to say that an important aspect of my own growth as a person and therapist is directly linked to the privilege that I have been given to journey along the road of recovery with the most affected survivors. It is difficult to quantify the immense courage they have shown in attempting to overcome their pain, and I share Zanarini's (2000) observation that they deserve to be congratulated for it. These issues are discussed in more depth in Part II of this book.

OBSERVATIONS BASED ON 180 SURVIVORS

This chapter concludes with the presentation of my own observations regarding the long-term effects of CSA. This information is presented in the form of categories referring to the survivors' coping level at presentation for therapy, and is organised in terms of their subjective report and my own observations in the early stages of therapy. The reader's attention is drawn to the fact that I make no particular claims about this information, other than pointing out that it is based on painstaking therapeutic application and observation over a decade's work. Moreover, the main aim of the presentation is to impart an integrated understanding of the issues that are central both to survivors' perception of their well-being and efficacy (or lack of it), as well as the therapist's own understanding. It is not within the scope or aim of the presentation to make definitive assumptions about causal factors—e.g. type of abuse, nature of perpetrator, etc.—although descriptions inevitably include this information. In keeping with the general ethos of the book, I considered it to be more relevant to focus on providing the reader with the clinical picture I have observed.

Category 1: "Coping very badly"

In the previous chapter I indicated that of the 180 women, thirty were considered to be coping very badly at initial presentation. What follows is a summary of the types of experiences that characterise their subjective report in terms of family background, sexual abuse, adolescence, and presenting problems.

Family environment

Accounts given allowed me to identify four general types of family environment: chaotic; unstable; incongruous; and emotionally inhibited.

Chaotic

This type is one where both parents or carers are living together, but where the atmosphere is one that inspires constant fear. Usually, one or both parents abuse alcohol and there is frequent domestic violence, both physical and verbal, usually towards the mother, leading survivors to feel responsible for the latter and in fear of losing her. Some survivors also experience physical violence from one or both of the parents and are regularly punished, criticised, or verbally humiliated. The survivors recall being unable to predict what would occur next, and living in constant fear that something terrible might happen. Their physical needs are neglected and they frequently have to assume responsibility for younger siblings. Typically, their schooling suffers as well as their social development, and they tend to leave home in mid-adolescence.

Unstable

Here, either mother or father has died or left the family home and the remaining parent finds it difficult to cope. Some survivors recall having been put into foster care for certain periods of time and then being taken back by their parent, usually the mother. Other survivors might have been placed in the care of grandparents or other close family members. Recollections include the parent as being vulnerable and unable to cope, being split up from siblings, a series of different men/lodgers coming into the house, feeling different to other children, confusion about who their primary carer is, lack of contact, and grief over the absent or dead parent.

Incongruous

Such families of origin are characterised by double standards. To the outside world they appear to be pillars of society, respectful of authority and public law, and are viewed as being highly disciplined. It is not unusual for these families to be church devotees, or to appear to uphold high moral codes of conduct. Behind closed doors this picture contrasts with lack of respect for personal boundaries, usually by the more dominant of the parents. Survivors have reported being verbally insulted and called names of a derogatory sexual nature, having comments made about their bodies, being accused of committing indecent acts, and never being allowed privacy. They have also expressed confusion about their parents' apparent contradictions, as well as not knowing how to behave. They also describe acute difference in parental power dynamics, with one being dominant, feared, and in some cases punitive as well as violent, and the other being submissive and unable to intervene. Survivors also recount their anger and disappointment at the fact that no one from the outside was able to notice or offer help when they themselves were being physically and/or sexually abused. What further characterises these families is their insularity from external influence and their active shunning of involvement from professional agencies.

Emotionally inhibited

For all intents and purposes, this is a "normal" type of family. The term "normal" is heuristic, and implies that the family is functioning reasonably well (according to external observation), and includes both-parent families, single parents, and reconstituted families. Although mostly self-sufficient and not usually involved with any type of helping or legal authority, what characterises this type of environment is its lack of appropriate emotional expression and recognition of the child's individual and nurturing needs. Survivors who described such experiences have expressed two types of situations. One is where there was a great deal of emphasis on achievement and success and the survivor felt that they were always falling short of expectation. Here, there is a tendency towards strict discipline and little positive reinforcement or affection. The other situation is where the survivor lacked guidance and perceived the parent or parents as being too distant or too absorbed in their own lives to pay attention to them. Indeed, survivors have frequently described their mothers as being either too inadequate or "absent" to attend to their needs and felt a constant yearning for attention.

It must be pointed out that these four categories are very broad and based on survivors' personal reports. The boundaries between them are quite arbitrary and any of them might share certain characteristics. Moreover, psychiatric illness, especially anxiety and depression in primary carers, and/or parental inadequacy was a recurring theme expressed by survivors, irrespective of family "category". However, the manner in which they are listed serves to highlight the most striking features of each of them in order to provide an appreciation of the survivors' early experience. This topic will be addressed in more detail in Chapter 13. Suffice it to say, that what unites all of the categories is their pervasive invalidating nature and neglect of survivors' emotional and psychological needs. Table 5.2 provides a summary of survivors' reports relating to abuse, adolescent experience, and presenting problems at initial therapeutic contact.

Discussion

The summary presented in Table 5.2 provides the most extreme "scenario" that I have observed in my involvement with female survivors of CSA. It must be noted that variations of this picture (i.e. not all features were necessarily present) was the case for thirty of the women, and to a slightly lesser extent for another fifty-five women whom I saw at the time of writing. What characterises the "coping very badly" group of survivors, and what differentiates them from other groups, relates to five factors:

- all of the women in this group had psychiatric histories;
- all of them expressed substantial difficulties in all of the following self-

Table 5.2 "Coping very badly": Broad history profile

Abuse characteristics	Adolescence	Presenting problems
Perpetrator: Likely to be a family member—namely father, stepfather (or mother's boyfriend), grandfather, brother, uncle. In two instances mother was an accomplice. A number of survivors in this group reported additional abuse from other figures outside the family home—e.g. neighbour, friend of the family.	**Reported features**: Perception of being different to peers; poor self-image; school bullying (mostly receptive); playing truant; poor educational achievement; delinquency; isolation and lack of peer support; alcohol/ substance abuse; self-mutilation; suicide attempts; assuming responsibility for siblings and/or parent; physical and/or emotional neglect; exposure to psychiatric and psychological services.	**Psychiatric**: Clinical depression; PTSD; obsessive compulsive disorder; anxiety; eating disorders; alcohol/drug addiction. **Psychological**: Low self-esteem; self-blame; depression; anxiety; agoraphobia; social anxiety; sexual problems; marital/relationship problems; parenting concerns; negative body image; lack of self-confidence; gender dysphoria.
Nature of abuse: All categories of abuse—i.e. I, C1, C2, and NC (see Chapter 4)—with the large majority reporting most categories at the hands of family carers and non-penetrative variations at the hands of most other abusers. However, not all survivors reported abuse involving penetration.		
Onset, frequency, and duration: Abuse usually starts well before puberty, it is likely to be carried out on a regular basis and over an extended period of time. Intercourse usually (but not always) stops during puberty.		**Behavioural**: Poor self-efficacy (e.g. home management, finances, parenting, employment); poor self-care; social avoidance; alcohol/ substance abuse; self-harm, suicidal attempts; revictimisation (i.e. domestic violence and/or sexual assault); poor communication skills and inability to have personal needs met; poor personal boundaries; aggression; mistrust; dependent and manipulative behaviour.

management areas: work, home, leisure, private and social, and relationships and communication;

- all exhibited traits that would be compatible with a diagnosis of borderline personality disorder;
- most had experienced incestuous abuse, particularly from fathers and father figures, in addition to other perpetrators in some cases;
- all of the women expressed issues related to all of Finkelhor's traumagenic dynamics.

The reader will have noted the absence of the survivors' emotional dimension in the summary table, but I wished to accord special attention to this. First of all I would like to convey that it is to these thirty women and also to those that were coping badly at presentation (see next category) that I owe the depth of my understanding of what it means to be sexually, as well as emotionally and psychologically abused. The intensity of their emotional pain, anger, and despair at what they perceived to be an uncaring, cruel, and abusing world, and their equally intense and desperate measures to deal with these feelings cannot fail but to deeply affect any therapist. Indeed, these women's presentations, at times, managed to throw into question a great deal of what I had learned and put me in the position of having to carefully revise not only my working practices (see Chapters 6 and 7) but also my preconceptions of human behaviour.

These survivors present with huge amounts of emotional baggage in many forms, including charm, seduction, dependency, anger, manipulation, and gratitude. The complexity of their difficulties is immense and requires the juggling of the psychiatric, emotional, behavioural, psychological, and social dimensions of their treatment. Their sense of powerlessness is acute and they adopt any means they can manage in order to maintain some semblance of life. Unfortunately, in the course of so doing they frequently manage to either alienate people further, including professionals, or indeed to perpetuate the invalidation they have previously experienced through abusive relationships. I am hugely indebted to these women not only because they have facilitated my own growth as a human being, but also because in helping them overcome their pain and achieve freedom from the past, I have experienced a personal and professional satisfaction that is proportional to the complexity of their case. What is more, it has confirmed to me that it is possible to transcend suffering and pain and that the term "survivor" is truly deserved.

Category 2: "Coping badly"

Fifty-five of the women who appeared to be coping badly at presentation for psychological treatment shared most of the features already discussed, particularly in terms of family background and type of perpetrator. A number of issues differentiate them, however, from those who were coping very badly. First, during their adolescent years they had fewer incidents of delinquency, suicide attempts, and less exposure to psychological intervention. They did, however, express problems in the other areas of adolescence mentioned in Table 5.2. Secondly, although most of the women had received psychiatric help in the past, this was less intensive and required fewer hospital admissions than the first group. Thirdly, the women in this group did not perceive themselves to have difficulties in all areas requiring daily management. For example, although they found employment difficult to sustain due to their anxiety and low self-esteem, some of them were able to manage their home and children, while others required the support of child and family services. By far the most common difficulty here concerned relationships, and this encompassed social, intimate, and family figures, especially mothers. The most striking feature uniting the women in this group (and those in the previous one) is their almost unanimous negative self-perception and stigmatisation. The latter was a deeply ingrained belief about their undesirability in many areas, including their intelligence and talents, physical looks, "personality" (i.e. they viewed themselves as boring, "no conversation", etc.), and most of all "unlovability". However, I found this never to be the case and indeed frequently found them to be the most intriguing, complicated, and kind individuals who would subjugate their needs to those of others in search of approval. When their anger and despair prompted unhelpful, angry, self-destructive, and manipulative behaviour, I found that appropriate confrontation and consistent boundary setting within a rubric of "limited parent", was rewarded by a determination to see the therapy through.

Categories 3 and 4: "Coping OK" and "coping quite well"

Survivors' initial presentation in these two categories (sixty and thirty-three survivors respectively) is in contrast to that of the two previous groups. This contrast, however, is mainly in terms of their subjective perception of coping with life's demands, but there are other differences which I shall address shortly. The women in this group tended to present with specific difficulties and had a reasonable clarity about which issues they wished to address in therapy. The latter revolved around problems with intimate relationships, including "marital" and/or sexual difficulties; request for guidance with ambivalent parental relationships, and in particular with mothers; low self-esteem; need for support during disclosure of the abuse; parenting concerns; and lack of direction and general dissatisfaction with life. Overall, however, the women who coped "quite well" in particular were able to hold down good jobs, manage their households, and have reasonable social lives. Indeed, to the outside world they were frequently perceived as being confident, able, and someone others could turn to for advice. That is not to say that they did not express deep unhappiness and bewilderment at their inability to find satisfaction in relationships and their tendency to repeat self-destructive patterns of behaviour about which they felt shame and disappointment. Indeed, it is not unusual for women in this category to seek referral for therapy when they realise that they are unable to sustain a relationship or during an episode of depression and/or acute anxiety, when they find themselves being confronted with issues in their past that they had managed to "put away". Other survivors in this group have sought help either following their own entry to motherhood, or when they were involved in a stable relationship. This makes it all the more distressing for them to try to understand why the past has come to haunt them, and I have devoted some discussion to this in Chapter 10.

In terms of other background characteristics, the women in these two groups had mainly experienced the "incongruous" and "emotionally inhibited" family background, although a few had had experience of the other two. Perpetrators of the abuse covered all types, although the general bias was towards "non-resident" family figures (related or otherwise) and also "strangers". The abuse started usually, but not always, during the early stages of puberty and tended to last for shorter periods than that for survivors in the "coping very badly/badly" categories. In contrast to the latter categories, the abuse was less frequent, over shorter periods of time, and quite often it occurred only "once or twice".

Other features noted in this group are worthy of some discussion. First, although some of the abuse details and family background in this group differed to that of survivors in the previous two categories, their pain and negative memories of their childhood was frequently as acute and disturbing. Secondly, in spite of the latter, the survivors in this group recalled themselves as having better self-efficacy and self-sufficiency during adolescence, and had experienced less school bullying, truancy, delinquency and had minimal exposure to professional agencies. Moreover, there was less alcohol and substance abuse, and substantially less self-harm than among the survivors in the first two groups. Thirdly, although the family background may have been cold, inhibited, or inconsistent, the survivors did recall instances of encouragement and guidance to succeed, and they were more likely to recall having had an emotional connection and support from a grandparent or other family figure. During adolescence, they were also more likely to belong to a stable peer group and have at least "one or two good friends". Fourthly and most importantly, although most did not express difficulties in all four traumagenic dynamics (see Finkelhor and Browne, 1986), almost all had issues with betrayal, not only related to the abuse, but mostly in terms of the lack of parental protection and ambivalent and/or invalidating reaction in instances when the abuse was disclosed.

Final comments

In presenting my own observations about the long-term effects of CSA, I have been acutely aware of the fact that our understanding about the specific variables that determine long-term adjustment or lack of it, is still in its infancy. It is for this reason that I have deliberately refrained from offering speculations about the links between certain abuse characteristics and particular sequelae. Having said this, in my view, the family of origin has been repeatedly shown to hold the utmost significance in relation to survivors' personal accounts about which issues were of most relevant concern to them. At the same time, the biosocial theory discussed in the previous section has much to offer, at least as an important adjunct to understanding individual differences. However, this theory too is far from being empirically validated.

Given these observations, it is hoped that the reader will appreciate the manner in which I have approached the presentation of the three case studies in Part II of the book. I have chosen a "narrative" style, in part, for three reasons:

1. I wanted to provide the reader with an opportunity to enter each of the survivor's worlds in order to gain an appreciation of their personal experience as well as an understanding of each of them as an individual.
2. I considered that the reader would gain a clearer and more relevant understanding of my stance regarding the integration of both theory and practice by providing an opportunity to view the issues raised in this chapter "in action".
3. Most importantly, I considered that the "narrative" style, as opposed to a more "reductionist" approach, would be a more appropriate medium in terms of ensuring the integrity and validation of survivors, and would remain faithful to the principles of the therapeutic relationship discussed in Chapters 6 and 7.

Part II

Integration, the alliance, and the therapist

Chapter 6

Model integration and therapeutic alliance

There is no such thing as a unique scientific vision, any more than there is a unique poetic vision. Science is a mosaic of partial and conflicting visions. But there is one common element in these visions. The common element is rebellion against the restrictions imposed by the locally prevailing culture.

Dyson (1995)

The second part of this book focuses on the intervention process and in this opening chapter I wish to introduce the areas, which, in combination, act as a guiding principle when I see survivors of sexual abuse. I discuss my reasons for adopting an "eclectic" stance when seeing survivors of sexual abuse — that is, by integrating two or more psychotherapeutic theories and/or techniques. The therapeutic alliance within this approach, I believe, is a central aspect of the intervention process, and in the second part of the chapter I present a brief overview of its historical significance with more emphasis on its importance in my own work.

MODEL INTEGRATION

In Chapter 1 I explained that I wished to present the material in this book in a manner that would convey the interactive nature of my work with survivors of sexual abuse. What I meant by this is that I wished to portray myself not as the "all knowing" and superior therapist imparting great theoretical knowledge or clinical expertise as a result of the work I have done, but as a person on an equal humanistic level with my patients, who is prepared to share the type of information about myself that can help the reader understand better how I evolved as a therapist. Hence, my discussion on why I opt for model integration will be clearer after I give a summary of my training background.

I trained in an environment that fosters a very high regard for objective and empirical methods and we were guided, from the early stages of our

training, to espouse a solid theoretical framework within which to formulate clinical problems and administer appropriate interventions. To some
this may seem a rather narrow and rigid approach, and there should always
(I believe) be a healthy degree of questioning and criticism of those who as
trainees are required to follow a rigid discipline. Looking back, I now feel
very indebted to this initial strict guidance as it has provided me with
an invaluable critical perspective, and has given me the basis of a sound
understanding of psychopathology and the means of assessing it. In my
opinion, however, I was still a "rebel", in that I was hungry to be exposed
to as many theoretical orientations as time could allow, and, in addition to
the intensive cognitive/behavioural training I received, I also added a year's
supervised training in psychodynamic therapy. This was extremely
enriching, not only because it provided what I considered to be a more
"rounded" exposure to different treatment approaches (during my under-
graduate years I had taken a particular interest in humanistic and gestalt
theories), but it also allowed me to examine the various criticisms adopted
by each "side of the fence", so to speak.

I have always considered myself to be primarily a clinician, in that I
derive the greatest satisfaction from being involved in the face-to-face
therapeutic situation. Having said this, the empirical part of my training
has acted as a conscience that calls upon me to examine and question the
particular route I might take with any individual I may be involved with.
This empirical conscience has led me to believe that the most important
aspect of learning about human beings and their difficulties, while building
on what I had learned as a trainee, was to be exposed to as much clinical
work as possible. The latter intention is one that I consider I am continuously addressing (having seen in excess of 2,000 patients in the past
twelve years), and it is this experience and the invaluable insights it has
afforded me which leads me to argue the following: A sound theoretical
basis is crucial but its therapeutic potential is limited if it excludes "competing" models that could be more appropriate for a particular individual
or, indeed, for a particular aspect of an individual's problem. Indeed, I
would go further to argue that a flexible and creative approach that integrates more than one model has greater potential.

Relational paradigms

This argument is one that is not without complexity and even controversy,
and it has been addressed by a number of writers (Abroms, 1983; Colapino,
1984; Safran et al, 1988). It is not within the scope and aims of this chapter
to develop an in-depth discussion on the issue but I will, nevertheless, refer
to some important arguments made by other writers as they have particular
relevance to the integrated approach adopted in this book. There are two
main propositions put forward by other writers, and while they may at first

glance appear to diametrically oppose the stance on eclecticism, they are nevertheless very pertinent to my own arguments. The first of these posits that it is not the particular theoretical framework or model adopted by a clinician that accounts for change but, rather that it is the non-specific quality of the therapeutic relationship which is responsible for this. This view was the result of a very much publicised paper, the methodology of which gained empirical credibility, and in which it was concluded that there were no differences in therapeutic outcome among the major schools of psychotherapy (Luborsky et al, 1975). The second argument is one that I find has qualified this premise in a manner supporting the view I hold regarding integration. In his opening comments, Rappaport (1991) high-lights the apparent contradiction between the Luborsky et al findings on the one hand, and the growing momentum in the adoption of eclecticism by psychotherapists of all schools. He cites as a cause for this growth the apparent discontent of psychotherapists in terms of the following: "Behav-ioural theory does not account for intrapsychic phenomena; psychoanalytic theory cannot adequately explain current social dynamic, cognitive theory has trouble explaining emotional phenomena, and virtually all therapy models cannot account for biological, gender, or cultural differences" (Rappaport, 1991, p. 165). The writer then develops the argument further by proposing that in fact the two "trends" are not necessarily oppositional, and contends that eclecticism does not imply a rejection of pure theoretical models, but of "relational paradigms" suggested by them.

The term "relational paradigm" is one that I refer to as the "the role of the therapist", and I discuss it in relation to myself in the next chapter. The manner in which Rappaport argues the pros and cons of the eclectic relational paradigm is in harmony with the manner in which I am attempt-ing to explain my reasons for integrating theories. A distinction is being made between eclectic relational paradigms and pure relational paradigms and Rappaport points to two main criticisms about the latter. First, that they have a limited scope—e.g. the psychoanalytic "blank screen" does not provide sufficient experiential parallels; client-centred approaches are not adequate for problem solving; and cognitive/behavioural theories do not address emotions. The second criticism (and this is one I have personally elaborated) is that pure relational paradigms do not have sufficient flexibility for application between clients and also within clients. That is, not all potential clients presenting for therapy are deemed "suitable", and also not all situations can be adequately addressed in the same client. The points made for the desirability of adopting an eclectic relational paradigm is therefore obvious, but it also has potential drawbacks. One of these rests on the premise that switching from one relational posture to another causes confusion for the client and may even arouse anxiety because there is no stable postural basis on which to modulate or "anchor" the relationship with the therapist. I agree wholly with this premise since it is compatible with my previous comments relating to the necessity of having a sound theoretical basis as well as extensive clinical experience before embarking on eclecticism. A further drawback (or at least necessity), Rappaport argues, is that while all practitioners must confront process values such as interpersonal qualities and therapeutic role, the eclectic therapist must be even more vigilant about these because there is no one particular stance that unites them all.

These are clearly very thought-provoking and pertinent observations for those choosing to adopt an eclectic relational paradigm and they must, therefore, be very carefully considered. In my case, I feel that I have overcome the potential dangers discussed by adopting the "limited re-parenting" paradigm. Indeed, I was very interested and even reassured to read (very recently) Rappaport's analysis of this as being the most effective basis on which to integrate therapeutic models and also relational stances. My adoption of this paradigm developed over the course of the early 1990s when I became very interested in schema-focused cognitive behaviour therapy (SFCBT), which, according to its developer (Young, 1994), is an integration of different theoretical models encompassing psychoanalytic, developmental, humanistic, and cognitive/behavioural perspectives.

Although this approach is an extension of Beck's cognitive behavioural therapy (CBT), because Young was one of the original associates in the initial publications of cognitive therapy, the writer later felt that CBT was not sufficient for addressing the types of difficulties that clients with personality difficulties, as a function of having experienced problematic childhoods, presented with. In particular, the acquisition of maladaptive schemas starting from a pre-verbal stage—such as "emotional deprivation", "defectiveness", "mistrust abuse", etc.—is considered to represent the central core of a person's subjective representation of life, particularly in terms of relationships with others. Factors relating to early emotional adaptation or lack of it due to maternal deprivation and quality of home environment, such as discussed by Bowlby (1973) and Winnicot (1965, 1986), are considered to be instrumental in the acquisition of personal schemas.

More recently, I was very encouraged to read a paper in *Behaviour Research and Therapy* (Arntz and Weertman, 1999) in which a very convincing argument was made about the importance of using experiential techniques in the treatment of childhood memories such as sexual abuse. The discussion was made against a backdrop of the work of professionals in the area of personality disorder (Pedesky, 1994), post-traumatic stress disorder (Smucker et al, 1995), and early maladaptive schemas (Young, 1994; McGinn and Young, 1996), who have all asserted the need for integrated approaches with these clinical presentations.

It has not really been my intention to promote or discuss the merits of SFCBT but I wanted to (a) provide a context within which to encapsulate my earlier discussion of eclecticism and theoretical integration and (b) to offer readers a signpost to Part III of the book on the therapeutic intervention that will illustrate the use of SFCBT with particular detailed reference to the case histories presented at the start of the book. It will become clear how this approach integrates all of the concepts I have described here (i.e. relational paradigms, theoretical framework, and intervention techniques). The concept of limited re-parenting and its therapeutic potential will be explained and discussed further when I address my role as therapist in the next chapter, and its relevance will be specifically illustrated in Chapters 9, 10, and 11. I must clarify at this point, however, that while schema-focused therapy provides a "central" basis or model from which to begin formulating and addressing problems, this does not exclude the use of other intervention techniques to be used when a specific difficulty needs particular intervention. I am referring here to techniques applied, for example, in couple therapy, sex therapy, addiction habits, phobias, etc., and that could be borrowed from a number of "theoretical schools" as deemed appropriate.

Relevance of model integration in the treatment of CSA

I would like to conclude this section by drawing together the various threads of its discussion with reference to survivors of sexual abuse, which was my primary aim of presenting it, especially in the light of the argument that a therapist's theoretical orientation can influence the manner in which the treatment of sexual abuse will be formulated and then addressed (Courtois, 1988). I maintain that, if this argument is correct, there will be pitfalls in the adherence to inflexible theoretical approaches and pure relational paradigms (or ways "of being" with a client), and these were discussed earlier. In my case, I have found that the immense complexity of the issues, difficulties, and distress that survivors of sexual abuse present with, as well as the spectrum of varying degrees of severity, cannot be responded to adequately by any one individual approach. The stories of three survivors of sexual abuse presented at the start of the book exemplify the types of difficulties the women can experience, and these do not, by any means, include all of the potential problems. The issues women wish to address can refer to a host of past, current, as well as future considerations, including the following:

- Specific resolution and "emotional processing" of the abuse itself.
- Understanding the family dynamics and part played by parents and/or carers in the past and also the present.
- Appreciation of the types of "templates" or "schemas" that are acquired during childhood and their role in maintaining maladaptive

patterns of behaviour, as well as repeating the cycle of abusive, neglectful, or abandoning relationships.

- Receiving practical and emotional support during the process of dealing with deliberate self-harm (i.e. self-mutilation) and/or dependence on alcohol and/or drugs.
- Dealing with problems of body image and maladaptive patterns of eating.
- The need to work towards autonomy and self-reliance in the present, and being guided in a practical manner in relation to issues such as the importance of the preservation of "personal boundaries", self-esteem, self-confidence, assertiveness, and personal resourcefulness.
- Understanding the implications of trust towards oneself and also others.
- Resolution of sexual difficulties on an individual and/or couple basis.
- Guidance and support when disclosing and confronting the abuse with families and perpetrators, and also when making official police statements, plus the implications of such actions.

This is certainly not an exhaustive list of the areas addressed during the course of therapy (discussed in more detail in the previous chapter), but they nevertheless clearly highlight the reasons for adopting an integrated intervention approach because the requirements for resolution are both abstract and specific. I also discussed the importance of professional responsibility when adopting eclecticism due to the potential confusion or anxiety a client may experience as a result of the "switching" to another relational paradigm. In view of this, I introduced the concept of limited re-parenting as an appropriate way of integrating various "ways of being", because the course of a parental role implies a variety of stances given a particular need for guidance, support, and encouragement. In addition, the limited re-parenting role within schema-focused CBT, with its acknowledgement of the influence of early environment, pre-verbal schema acquisition, faulty and/or abusive relationships, emotional factors, and maladaptive behaviour as potential modulators of personality and relational difficulties, succeeds, in my opinion, in consolidating my empirical as well as professional principles when helping people. Most crucially, I have found that this approach shifts the focus from pathologising survivors of sexual abuse, because faulty schema acquisition has a dimensional quality along which anyone may hold a place. Implied in this approach is the emphasis on the collaborative relationship, whether one is addressing the here and now or "processing" past events. I would argue further that in my case I have found that therapeutic alliance or relationship lies at the heart of my work with survivors of sexual abuse and, for this reason, I am introducing it in the next section and will follow this with a separate chapter on the personal characteristics and responsibilities I consider have been most relevant in my clinical practice.

THE THERAPEUTIC ALLIANCE

A great deal has been written in recent years about the therapeutic alliance or relationship, mostly within the domain of counselling psychology, but its role has also been discussed in relation to cognitive therapy and I will be referring to some of this work. I consider, however, that other clinicians reading this book might appreciate the additional personal focus of my own experience and I will expand on this (in the next chapter), after providing an overview of the historical and current perspective regarding the therapeutic relationship.

The concept of "therapeutic relationship" is one that, while it is probably considered central to most face-to-face interactions between therapist and client, is also one that is taken for granted with little apparent specification of its exact role within the therapeutic process. This criticism is one that has been mostly meted out to the more behavioural and even cognitive psychotherapies, although I shall be referring to some recent publications that dispute this notion. Historically, the therapeutic dyad has been mainly the domain of psychoanalytic, psychodynamic and, a little later, counselling therapies. In the first two, the process of transference and counter-transference acts as a core mediating process between the patient's intrapsychic events and the therapist's own interpretation and reflection, with a view to resolution via insight.

In counselling psychotherapies, initially led by the writings of Carl Rogers, the emphasis has been on humanistic variables such as empathy, warmth, acceptance, and the potential for personal growth. The advent of radical behaviourism in the early part of this century and the development of allied psychotherapies with their emphasis on empiricism, appeared to pay little attention to the part played by the therapist in terms of his/her particular personal characteristics. This apparent gulf between the schools of psychotherapy mentioned and those based on behaviourism has been related to the fact that the first acknowledged the part played by emotions in the patient's distress, while the latter approach appeared to deny the existence of these because the principles of therapy where primarily based on cause and effect paradigms founded on classical and operant conditioning and, later, learning theories (Pavlov, 1927; Skinner, 1938; Wolpe, 1958, 1969; Eysenck, 1960).

Starting in the 1960s, Aaron Beck's work linking thinking processes with depression (1963, 1964, 1967) heralded a revolution in its application within clinical psychology, and the academic as well as clinical publications continue to dominate in this field. In particular, the work of Beck and his associates (Beck 1976; Beck et al, 1979) has provided the cornerstone of CBT interventions for the first instance treatment of depression. Its empirically documented success in treating this condition has extended its application to most other adult clinical complaints.

The application of CBT relies on a collaborative relationship between clinician and patient, and although this has gone some way towards acknowledging the importance of a therapeutic relationship, this has not totally appeased the criticism by sceptics of CBT. More recently, however, the work of therapists in the currently growing area of counselling psychology has contributed important insights to the debate about the therapeutic relationship in general (Feltham, 1999) and its importance in CBT in particular (Wills and Sanders, 1997; Sanders and Wills, 1999). Sanders and Wills (1999) provided a very illuminating analysis about the therapeutic relationship by reviewing the literature on it, and also by drawing on the work of Safran (1990) and Safran and Segal (1990), who have provided an important examination of the therapeutic role in CBT. The summary of the combined arguments is that CBT and the more extended SFCBT have a dimensional perspective whereby specific and easily solvable problems are addressed via a collaborative relationship within a problem-solving context (in the first), while more complex difficulties involving faulty relationships and "problems" of the self that are mediated by emotions need to be addressed within a more dynamic therapeutic relationship. The main argument to be derived from these writers is that CBT may have been unfairly judged and that, while it has at one end of the spectrum a very practical ethos that apparently denies the role played by emotions, this is not its only application because emotions, indeed, are acknowledged as the spectrum progresses towards more complex difficulties (Young, 1994; Safran, 1996).

So what is my own experience as a clinical psychologist in terms of my role as a therapist? Although female survivors of sexual abuse do not constitute my sole client group, and even though I aspire to certain values and principles when seeing all my patients, my experience with survivors of abuse has had an instrumental impact on my mode of practice, with them in particular, but also in general.

What I have been made distinctly aware of is that "listening" to survivors in the first instance is the only way in which they will become engaged in their therapy. The spectrum of potential needs as described earlier is very pertinent here, and I accord the necessary respect to my clients by allowing them to define the issues they wish to address. I have also been made aware that, whether we like it or not, people presenting for therapy are consumers as they would be in any other area of life that offers commodities and, mostly, they are in the position of knowing what they would like and need. Following on from this argument, if a survivor of sexual abuse comes to see me and asks me to help her with certain practical issues such as learning to deal better with an overpowering boss, social anxiety, or general stress, then this is what I must respond to. I may of course have my own formulation about the possible relevance of these problems in terms of the overall history of abuse in early childhood, but consider that it would be counter-productive to suggest that all these issues will naturally resolve once the "underlying" problem is addressed. To do so would, in my opinion, further disempower the woman and might even alienate her from returning to therapy, and would also communicate a lack of empathy towards the problems that she considers to be important to her. In other words, by responding in a collaborative and respectful manner, I can begin to impart the feeling that we may become equal partners in a relationship aimed at resolving difficulties. It could be the case that once certain practical issues have been addressed the survivor perceives herself to be "well" and does not choose to return for the more in-depth resolution of the abuse, and, in such circumstances, I have to accept this is a choice she has made, while at the same time keeping "the door" open should she wish to return. This very frequently happens and so I feel I have provided the necessary trust and safety that enables some survivors to regulate the pace of their therapy. As I mentioned in Chapter 4, the nature of the environment in which I work affords the possibility of "paced" therapy continuity, which I think is very advantageous.

Another crucial issue I have been made aware of when working with survivors of sexual abuse is the importance of "validating" their disclosures. Of course, all of our patients are concerned that we may not understand, believe, or appreciate the extent of their distress, but in the case of survivors of abuse I would assert that being believed or validated is paramount for them. I have derived this understanding by noting that the secrecy that is an endemic part of the state of having been abused constitutes, arguably, one of the main negative maintaining factors of the ongoing distress the women complain of. Keeping the abuse secret is the unspoken, or most frequently, coerced rule by which perpetrators ensure that their acts are not uncovered. When I say "unspoken" I am referring to the survivors' distress when as adults they do not comprehend why they were unable to tell of their ordeal. After all, they say, "I was not threatened with my life", or "I was not subjected to violence or pinned down", and "yet I felt as though I could not tell anyone, because I did not know how to and also I was afraid I would not be believed, even though I knew something not right was being done to me".

When secrecy is imposed through coercion by psychological means, a perpetrator will typically say things like, "no one will believe you" and then follow this by threats of potential consequences such as, "you will be put in a home"; "the family will have to break up", "everyone will hate you", and so on. Under these circumstances, disclosure presents a very grave risk to survivors (even disclosure to a therapist) due to the long-standing duration of the internalised secret world of the abuse and the perceived dangers of disclosure. The importance of not only validating the survivors' experience, but of doing this in a manner that can begin to provide the necessary safety within which to break the silence which then facilitates the progress of therapy, I believe, constitutes the primary concern of the therapeutic alliance. After all, if survivors do not trust us and if they feel unable to relate to us, how or why should they tell us anything? Indeed, I would go one step further and argue that my own experience of working with survivors of sexual abuse approximates to the analogy of "going on a journey" in which there is an element of the unknown and where I perceive myself as a "guide" who, while in possession of the map, nevertheless can be subject to climatic and topographical variations. Using this analogy, the importance of the therapeutic alliance for me is paramount beacuse, unless I am trusted to act as a skilful and competent guide as well as one who will appreciate the potential difficulties my "walkers" may have to face, then they may abandon the trek well before we reach the summit. On the other hand, I need to be skilful in my recognition that "walkers" come with different levels of ability and fitness and that I must be responsible enough to guide each of them within the limits of their own wishes and abilities.

The latter observation is one that has been very instrumental in shaping some of the personal characteristics, or "ways of being", that I adopt in the therapeutic alliance. In the next chapter I discuss and illustrate in more detail my personal stance and the attitudinal "philosophies" that I observe, and which have been influenced by other therapists.[1]

Chapter 7

Therapists' personal characteristics and roles: My experience

This chapter is an extension of the previous one and here I would like to consolidate and also illustrate some of the issues that were raised there, particularly in terms of "ways of being" within the therapeutic alliance and also the "relational paradigms" or therapeutic roles. To make this more explicit in terms of my work with survivors of sexual abuse, I have divided the chapter into two sections. The first deals with the variables or personal characteristics that I am continually attempting to develop and internalise to greater effectiveness; the second section outlines the primary roles or responsibilities I have learned are essential when helping survivors to work through their experience of sexual abuse.

PERSONAL CHARACTERISTICS: A PERSON-CENTRED APPROACH

> The person-centred approach is not a psychology, a psychotherapy, a philosophy, a school, a movement nor many other things frequently imagined. It is merely what its name suggests, an *approach*. It is a psychological posture, a way of being, from which one confronts a situation.
>
> (Wood, 1996, p. 161)

This quotation succinctly describes my belief about the essence of person-centred variables as discussed extensively by Carl Rogers (1951, 1957, 1959, 1980). There is an important distinction to be made, however, in terms of the variables' mediating purpose within therapy, as adopted by Rogers on the one hand and other clinicians on the other. I personally subscribe to the belief that the person-centred variables (which I will discuss below) are essential in facilitating as well as enhancing the process of therapy and, as such, they are not therapeutic tools. Rogers' belief, however, was that if the necessary conditions were present, such as congruence, empathy, and unconditional positive regard, this alone would enable the client to find his/her own answers to their difficulties through the process of "self-actualisation".

My own argument is that people who come to us for help need not only our acceptance, understanding, and honesty, but they also expect that we will help and guide them towards a resolution of their problems. That is not to say that they do not have the capacity to find their own answers, as mostly they do, but when the pattern of their life has been disrupted and unhelpful vicious circles have been created, it is our responsibility to take an active part in redressing some of these acquired patterns. This is a great task indeed, particularly when the problems are complex and diverse. In summary, my experience of working with a great number of adult women who were sexually abused in childhood has brought to my attention the need to be flexible and creative by adopting an eclectic approach to therapy through model integration rather than particular model rejection. At the same time, it is important for me to be able to be competent and communicate to my clients a sense of confidence and stability in what I do, and this I address by adopting the relational paradigm of "limited parent". This paradigm, or stance, affords me both the necessary flexibility (because parents need to adopt different approaches for any given problem) and also the anchor with which to stabilise the different approaches.

Working with survivors of sexual abuse has, in addition, had a fundamental influence on my personal presentation as a practitioner because I have been made aware that my general manner, demeanour, and verbal interaction can be of great significance in the development of a positive therapeutic relationship. Survivors frequently describe their distress in terms of "faulty" relationships they have experienced both in childhood and also later in life, and so they are particularly sensitive and sharply perceptive about how others relate to them. Through the process of my own development and learning during the course of my work I have been repeatedly drawn towards the writings of Rogers as I found myself progressively regulating my "way of being" according to his principles; when adopting them my experience and, I believe my patients' experience, was enriched as a result. In this sense, the continual refining of my personal presentation is an ongoing process (no one reaches perfection!) that envelops and guides me during the process of therapy, but it is not expected to fulfil the actual demands of intervention. This, at least, is my position based on personal experience and, for obvious reasons, it is not one that could be subjected to empirical scrutiny. I am merely describing what I have found works best during the therapeutic journey the survivors and I embark on when they seek my help.

The following discussion looks more closely at the person-centred variables I aspire to and attempt to adopt.

Congruence

Congruence or genuineness is one of the three basic variables that Rogers hypothesised as being central to counselling. More specifically, he believed that a person's personal growth was facilitated by the therapist's ability to be honest and without "front" or façade. In my work with survivors of sexual abuse, this is a particularly important issue. In the previous chapter I introduced the concept of personal schemas or templates that people acquire during the course of their childhood and how some of these schemas can be unhelpful in later life. One such schema relates to feelings of mistrust and suspicion towards people, which when looked at closely appears to originate from the experience of abuse at the hands of previously trusted family members or friends.

Women with a mistrusting "template" by which to make sense of the world develop a very keen sense of assessing people's level of honesty as well as motives. Consequently, when faced with a therapist whom they may perceive as being unapproachable or lacking in genuine qualities, they may well flee from the therapy. When survivors of sexual abuse present in a manner that conveys lack of trust, suspiciousness, fear, or inability to engage, then the genuineness with which the therapist promptly addresses this is very important in conveying honesty.

Another schema or template may refer to feelings of defectiveness or not being "good enough". In such a situation, a perception on the part of the patient of the apparent aura of the therapist as indicating superiority due to a starchy professional manner may reinforce her feelings of inadequacy and low self-worth due to a perceived overwhelming inequality. Congruence here could represent a very important first impression helping to lend to the return and engagement of the patient. I personally believe that a professional manner is exemplified by the level of integrity and responsibility towards one's task and not by a distant, authoritarian, or clinical manner. A particular encounter with one survivor brought this notion home to me in a most emphatic manner and I am indebted to her for giving me the opportunity, very early in my career, of reviewing my "way of being". A young woman came to see me because she wanted to discuss the gradual deterioration of her relationship with her partner, which she attributed to the fact that she was sexually abused as a child by her uncle. When she came to my room she appeared very tense and gave the impression of being very ill at ease, and she sat very stiffly on the edge of her chair throughout the session. She did not smile once, but was able to answer clearly and coherently the questions I asked, although I detected a great reluctance on her part to elaborate on any of her answers. I gave her a further appointment and did not give my own presentation a second thought, because I considered that I was by nature a caring and dedicated clinician, and I attributed her general demeanour to the fact that it must have been very difficult for her to address an issue that was clearly causing her pain.

It was only in retrospect, and after I received a letter from her (for which I am very grateful indeed) that I realised that her discomfort lay with the fact that she perceived me as cold and "clinical", and that I was more interested in "collecting facts" through the use of questionnaires (this in effect related to one questionnaire only) and she would have preferred to speak to a more accessible, "real person". She also said that she would not return to see me and that she would seek another, more approachable therapist. I remember when I first read this letter experiencing a host of emotions, not least that of rejection. At first I was bemused, because I considered myself totally devoted to my work, then angry at being so misunderstood, and finally sought comfort in the convenient belief that she was probably "not ready to work through her difficulties". But my inner conscience would not allow me to let the matter rest and I read and reread the letter countless times in an attempt to enter the experience of this young woman who had found me so unapproachable and who, as a result, did not wish to see me again.

When I understood and processed the impact of her letter on me, I replied to it and I believe that my reply marked an important realisation: that it is not sufficient to believe that one is a caring and genuine practitioner who only has the client's best interests at heart. It is vital that one is also vigilant to the manner in which this is portrayed, and that personal values such as congruence, and the ease with which we are able to be perceived as real people, are under constant examination. I exercised this revelation by replying with honesty and saying that she had brought to my attention some very important issues and that I was sorry she had experienced her session so negatively. I was also comfortable in saying to her that her observations had been taken on board and thanked her for her own willingness to share her impressions with me.

This particular encounter gave me the additional insight that it is more important to listen to what survivors have to say and not be distracted by technical aspects such as the handing out of questionnaires. Another issue here relates to an imbalance of perceived "power". Survivors always refer to the fact that they were powerless to exert any changes during the time they were abused and so they can be very uneasy if they perceive that their encounter with a therapist activates feelings of submission. By being congruent, a therapist would address such a potential perception very early on by reflecting their feelings of what may be going on: for example, "I feel as though you are tense and finding it difficult to tell me more about what is troubling you. Is there something about the way in which I am asking you questions or about me which makes this difficult for you?" I have found that this direct approach can produce a significant shift in the interaction between the survivor and myself because it succeeds in breaking any potential deadlock and also it asserts to her the fact that I am not just a therapist but a human being who is comfortable about questioning my own actions. To illustrate congruence further, some words from Wilkins (1999) approximate to my own beliefs about it: "Congruence (also referred to as genuineness or authenticity) is the quality of harmony between a person's inner experiencing and their outward expression. . . . The counsellor's congruence dissipates professional mystique and facilitates movement towards an egalitarian relationship" (Wilkins, 1999, p. 58–59).

The issue of self-disclosure in relation to congruence is frequently queried by people when I present workshops, and here I need to explain that congruence does not imply self-disclosure (Mearns and Thorne, 1988). I need to consider carefully how self-disclosure would affect the process of therapy because it is my primary concern that I do the best I can by my client and not use her to offload my feelings. Doing so would have several negative outcomes: the disclosure may overwhelm my client; it may perpetuate feelings of subjugation in her, since she may feel that the focus has been taken away from her; she may feel manipulated; and/or the disclosure may trigger feelings of guilt that her problems may not be so great after all. Therefore, I follow the rule that self-disclosure is only used when there is absolute confidence that this is done to facilitate the process or resolution of a particular issue during the course of therapy.

There could be said to be two types of self-disclosure: one that relates to the feelings I have about my client and the other to experiences I have had in my own life. If we take the first, would I be incongruent if I did not communicate feelings of irritation, anger, or boredom towards my client? My own approach to this is that I would have to be very in tune about the reasons that are making me feel this way (i.e. counter-transference), and then communicate them in such a manner that they are not perceived as critical or rejecting, but as helpful observations. For example, I was seeing a woman who was very consistent with her appointments and maintained that the therapy was helping her, and yet she usually spoke very little and I was becoming aware that I was doing most of the talking and being very directive. I was starting to get feelings of frustration as her few responses appeared to be motivated mostly by compliance and not collaboration and so I said to her, "I have noticed that I am the one who usually does the talking and I sometimes feel like a teacher who is not sure where her pupil is and what she is thinking, can you help me understand why I should feel this way?" The result of this reflection was quite dramatic in that she started to cry and said that before I said this to her she had assumed that she was there to follow my instructions and that no one usually asked for her opinion. In fact, she was not at all sure why she was there because it was her referrer who had suggested she seek help, but that she would now like to explore why she was unable to have confidence in her own opinions and feelings.

With respect to self-disclosure about personal issues, I may do this at a very much later stage in therapy, and only when the motive is clearly one of helping or inspiring the patient, rather than a reason with which to engage her. I will also try to be as "helpfully" honest when asked a direct question, such as, "have you ever been depressed", to which I might reply, "Yes, I have known depression"—but without elaborating further if I am not asked. The reason for this, in my view, is that patients come in a state of wanting to talk about and disclose matters of great personal importance to them and, therefore, the primary focus should be on them and they must not be distracted or preoccupied by issues in the therapist's life. Overall, by being congruent I will only self-disclose issues of a personal nature in terms of two rules: first, will this disclosure aid the progress of my patient, and secondly, do I feel comfortable in making this disclosure? I can say with some confidence that this issue has never been problematic because I have never felt the need to "lean on my patients", nor have they ever asked questions that threatened my integrity in any way. In my experience, I have found that the process of mutual respect has never been compromised, and this has not diminished my personal comfort in being as "real" a person as possible within the therapeutic alliance.

Empathy

An empathic understanding of the patient's private world is another valued characteristic that I aspire to within the therapeutic alliance. Empathy must be differentiated from sympathy, or simply expressing understanding of what someone relates to us, because these two qualities alone may convey a patronising stance. Empathy, on the contrary, is the ability to put oneself totally in the "other person's shoes", so to speak, as if the meaning of the person's experience is our own. According to Rogers, it is the "as if" quality that is of importance here and refers to the ability to listen to and to appreciate a person's anger, fear, emotional pain, or disillusionment without becoming engulfed by these feelings. When a therapist has an empathic appreciation of the client's world and feels at ease about moving within it freely, this creates a situation whereby he/she can communicate meanings that can facilitate the client's own understanding and acceptance of their experience. It is such a condition that can facilitate the gaining of insight and change.

Being truly understood by another human being is a very powerful and significant experience for anyone, and to be able to communicate empathic understanding towards someone who has seldom experienced this can open many doors for them, not least the courage to face up to past demons. While working with survivors of sexual abuse I have become aware of some common experiences they share, such as the feeling of alienation from others and thinking that they are "different" and at times even "defective". Other feelings relate to self-alienation and not having a clear identity. Fear can be a great part of survivors' experience in that they become hyper-vigilant to certain situations and are frequently on their guard as they expect the worst to happen. The issue of trust can, for survivors, be at best an alien concept, and at worst something that cannot be contemplated, even towards oneself. Being empathic towards these very complex emotions is indeed a challenge because frequently they are not verbally communicated, but are evident in the general presentation of survivors. Empathy in this sense is not just a simple act of "listening", but a more profound transpersonal process that involves physiological, perceptual, and verbal modalities. For example, it is not unusual for me to sense the fear or anxiety that a survivor is feeling when she enters my room for the first time. It is something I can almost experience in a physical way, possibly due to a sudden surge of adrenaline or discomfort in myself. It is not something that I can explain using specifics, only that it is my "own feeling" that is communicated through the client's own general demeanour. Because I am familiar with such a feeling I am not overwhelmed by it and I address it in a way that helps the survivor to feel validated and understood.

Learning to be empathic may appear to be an unattainable goal, and it is true that it is extremely difficult to achieve. Being able to be truly empathic is not a gift accorded to special people only; it can be achieved through hard grafting and a genuine willingness to commit time and effort. Empathy can best be described as a quality that belongs to the very human aspect of our being, and while it may be viewed as rather abstract it can be learned and developed. Certainly, it requires that the person is prepared to become acquainted with themselves in an honest manner via self-observation and, even better, through the experience of personal therapy.

In my experience, the ability to be empathic developed mostly from a very deep wish to understand the experience of those who were sexually abused as well as the experiences of my other patients. There is a continual process of trial and error as well as constant vigilance (to this day) about how best to listen, observe, and understand, and also to be honest about my own failings and be prepared to address them. The feedback survivors give me is possibly the most significant guidance I have about what I am trying to achieve, and this feedback has been the main encouragement I have received in my work. I once summarised to a survivor my understanding of her situation as follows: "I sense that you must be feeling so alone and isolated and this feels very sad and even frightening. You have a deep need to be loved and accepted, yet what you tell me says that people in the past were more interested in getting what they could from you rather than listening to what you want. So, although you want to be close to people, you feel you must keep away from them. It feels as though there is no way out". This reflection prompted the feedback; "You have put this better than I ever could—this is exactly how it feels and I would like to find a way out". To me, this simple feedback is the most powerful guidance I could ever need.

In Rogers' philosophy, empathy can promote change and growth within the individual by acting as a basis from which the client finds his/her own answers. I would go further and suggest that when clients perceive the empathic appreciation of their therapist, this creates a trusting and mutually respectful alliance within which the therapist's guidance is seen as offering viable avenues of choice towards the enhancement of well-being and independence. I have already referred to the fact the most survivors of sexual abuse primarily seek validation of their experiences and feelings, and it is crucial that this validation is achieved early on. I find that remaining alert to the importance of empathy means that the journey towards recovery becomes established and the setbacks or difficult climbs are more effectively managed.

Positive regard

The third therapist variable that completes my basic ethos of how "to be" with patients is that of having positive regard for them. In his initial written contributions, Rogers advocated "unconditional positive regard", which is characterised by a total acceptance and respect of the individual without conditions. I feel sceptical about this proposition, and Rogers, in one of his later contributions expressed his reservations about the unconditional aspect of regard (Rogers and Stevens, 1973). My own reservations refer first to the idea that we may accept a person with unconditional respect, but surely we would forfeit the first premise of congruence if we did not reflect on particular behaviours on the part of a patient, if this was considered to be unhelpful, contradictory, or self-destructive. I consider this premise to be compatible with my belief that we all deserve respect for our individuality as human beings, but that our behaviour may not always be desirable or compatible with our beliefs. Secondly, my experience in treating survivors of sexual abuse suggests that almost always there was either an absence of appropriate parental guidance, or by contrast, there existed a lack of individual respect towards the patient, within a context of a very harsh and unreasonably strict environment. I believe, therefore, that while positive regard for the individual is important, at the same time it is also a vital aspect of my role to point out and guide this individual as appropriate, remaining alert to respect and empathy. This point will be made clearer in the next section when my role as therapist will be discussed.

Positive regard then, is the variable that refers to the ability of showing warmth and acceptance towards the individual in a non-possessive manner. This appears to allow the survivor to feel that they are able to be open about their experiences without the fear of judgement or reprimand. Non-verbal cues, such as facial expressions and bodily posture are as important as the words used, because they can convey quite powerfully to the client what the therapist feels or thinks. I remember clearly one time when a survivor was reading out to me an account of her abuse experience, and she would frequently look up towards me. When she finished she said to me: "I am so grateful you sat so calmly and relaxed while I was reading because I was afraid you would find what I was saying too strange and disgusting and that you would tense up, become angry or worry: this would have made me stop".

What is described here is something which I am sure we are all aware of and which our experience has automatically internalised. I am also only too aware, however, of the fact that as human beings, we are subject to the pressures of clinical work and other pressures in general, and that with all the best intentions we may convey irritation, impatience, fatigue, or become distracted without even realising it. In my experience, when this has happened momentarily, it made me aware of the importance of not only reflecting this lapse of attention with the patient, but also of being vigilant in the future. Finally, positive regard communicates itself genuinely only when it is inspired by a deep belief in the respect of human individuality and not when it is couched in a belief of social desirability, or a paternalistic stance.

Summary

In this first section of the chapter I have discussed the variables that I have found to be important for the therapeutic alliance with survivors of sexual abuse. Although the importance of these variables has been emphasised within the context of such work, this does not imply that I do not observe them with other patients, but that it has been brought to my attention that vigilance about their application is particularly pertinent in the work with survivors of sexual abuse. I have discussed the characteristics that relate to congruence, empathy, and positive regard, and that while these are inspired by the extensive work of Carl Rogers, they are not adopted as a primary vehicle for change in any one individual. This is in stark contrast to Rogers who hypothesises that change follows naturally when such variables are at play due to their ability to create the necessary conditions for individuals to find their own answers. The reasons for remaining vigilant to them, in my own experience, is because I have found that when I do so a positive, trusting, and collaborative therapeutic alliance is formed and maintained, and this facilitates engagement and the progress of therapy, but I dispute the fact that they alone instigate change. The reason for this is that when an individual has lacked appropriate guidance in childhood and when this is combined with the experience of abuse, be it sexual, physical, or psycho-logical (in any combination), as well as neglect, then the therapist has a duty to be an active guide towards the resolution of problems that survivors present with. The variables relating to congruence, empathy, and positive regard are not, as such, therapeutic techniques, but personal characteristics that have the potential to communicate the first message of respect towards a survivor of sexual abuse, as well as the validation of their experience. At the same time, it must be pointed out that I agree with Rogers that all three variables, while aspired to and at times fulfilled, are extremely difficult to perfect and observe at all times and with everyone. They also require relentless practice.

MY ROLE AND RESPONSIBILITIES AS THERAPIST

In the final part of this chapter I discuss what I have experienced as being my role when seeing female survivors of sexual abuse. I should point out that the various areas of responsibility outlined are not the product of specific theoretical constructs, but have evolved and become established during the course of my involvement with survivors of sexual abuse. There exists, in addition, a large body of literature relating to this topic should the reader wish to have a wider perspective (Courtois, 1988; Sanderson, 1990; Kirschner, Kirschner, and Rappaport, 1993; Roth, 1993).

Providing safety and trust

It is of great importance to create a safe and trusting environment for survivors of sexual abuse. I see this as my initial responsibility, because unless the survivor feels that she is comfortable and at ease she will not easily engage with me let alone disclose very intimate and painful material. On the face of it, this appears to be an easy enough goal to achieve, but attention to detail is the key to creating the comfort and trust needed. In doing so, both the physical aspects of the therapeutic environment are important, as well as the physical and interpersonal characteristics of the therapist. With respect to the first, one must bear in mind that a great number of professionals conduct their clinical work in hospitals, day centres, or other therapeutic venues where there is limited scope for physical manipulation of a particular room. I am fortunate in that in my current practice (although not private) I have my own room, which is spacious and where I have reasonable scope for creating a personal atmosphere. Although it contains various books, journals, a personal computer, etc., which clearly define the room as an office, these are not, in my view, imposing in a manner that could alienate a particular client into feeling intimidated by a perception of the room being too cold or clinical, or because it may highlight perceived feelings of inadequacy. This is particularly so, because the room also contains some items suggesting certain aspects of my own individuality, such as postcards, pictures, a few photographs, and so on. In my view, a relaxed, warm atmosphere, which is both professional as well as suggesting that the therapist is comfortable being themselves (while not overpowering the client with their own private lives and preferences), can create the first impression of ease which in turn can facilitate engagement. In addition to these observations, appropriate seating arrangements conforming to the general rules for comfort and "power dynamics" are also important.

Another relevant observation I feel I should make is that my room is situated within an outpatient psychiatric department and, although the psychology department of which I am a member is constitutionally separate, my patients nevertheless need to use the same waiting room. Although some of the women who I see and who also happen to have contact with psychiatry do not have negative feelings about the use of this waiting room, those who are self-referred or referred from different agencies sometimes do. I am sure other professionals must be faced with such a situation, and in my case I have tried to minimise any discomfort, firstly by mentioning the sharing of the waiting room by more than one department in the appointment letter, and also by addressing it at the first session if I detect that this is an issue for a particular women or if, indeed, she mentions it herself. This example is one that highlights both the physical and inter-personal aspect of initiating a safe and trusting environment, by taking on board the issue of a client's first impressions and by acknowledging any potential discomfort. Other aspects relating to the physical environment are general "common sense" issues, such as avoiding all interruptions (i.e. by placing a sign on the door), avoiding extremes of temperature, ensuring that the environment is quiet, and, of course, that telephone calls are not being answered during sessions. Such measures may impart very early on a feeling within the survivor that she is important and respected.

The initial meeting with a survivor may be instrumental in terms of whether or not she will engage with the therapist. The level of comfort, safety, and trust a woman experiences during her first appointment may well have a direct bearing as to whether she will return. In addition to aspects relating to the physical environment, the therapist's personal char-acteristics are equally, if not more, pertinent. In the preceding section, the variables relating to congruence, empathy, and positive regard were dis-cussed. It is particularly important to be vigilant to those characteristics at the initial stages of the assessment and therapeutic interaction because they are directly relevant in terms of building mutual respect and understanding, thereby creating a safe and trusting foundation on which to build. More specifically, active listening that is totally focused on the survivor is my primary goal. Although I need to make notes for history taking and signposting purposes, I ensure that this does not conflict with providing undivided attention, even if it means completing my notes immediately after the session. I also explain the reasons why I have to make notes, but emphasise that confidentiality is always observed and that no one has access to my notes unless permission is given. Although active listening may be considered a relatively simple rule to observe, in my experience one can easily become distracted or sidetracked by wishing to formulate too early a particular problem, or by relying too heavily on theoretical constructs for guidance during the initial stages of therapy. I have to admit it is a skill that I have improved over the years because the feedback I receive from women, be it verbal or non-verbal, is that total empathic and non-judgemental attention to what a survivor says is the key to engagement. It must not be forgotten that most survivors will have seldom disclosed their experience of abuse in much detail.

They arrive at their first appointment with feelings of great trepidation, embarrassment, and fear of rejection or ridicule. It is very common for women whom I meet for the first time to say, "I'm so nervous being here, I feel so embarrassed of talking about what happened. It is so awful, and I'm scared of going back to those terrible memories". When survivors harbour such feelings—and the majority do—listening with patience, empathy, and non-judgementally is crucial, as is adopting an alert yet relaxed posture, with good eye-contact that is not threatening or distant, but warm. These characteristics ensure that trust and safety are present and this context can signal the start of self-validation for the survivor. Another important factor to be borne in mind is that survivors present with a variety of feelings, and at times (even at a first consultation) their expressions of anger, disappoint-ment, or total hopelessness may be very evident and even directed at the therapist. It is the therapist's responsibility to be mindful of creating the appropriate environment, and to appreciate the process of transference and counter-transference that is in operation and deal with this sensitively and competently in order to maximise the likelihood that the patient will return.

Last but by no means least, the therapist's personal attitudes, particularly in relation to sexuality, sexual abuse, and child abuse in general, must not impinge on the therapeutic alliance. This area of work can be a very distressing one due to the many stories a therapist will hear of the pain and endurance of survivors when they were children, and in many cases the sexual difficulties they experience as adults. A therapist should not only be empathic, but must also be aware of their own sexual history and attitudes, as well as their attitudes to "distasteful" behaviour in others, such as perpetrators of child abuse. Survivors are very vigilant of a therapist's reaction, be it verbal or non-verbal, to the disclosures they make and, therefore, before embarking on working with survivors of sexual abuse, every therapist has a duty to deal with his/her own personal agenda in terms of these issues and must also remain equally vigilant to any counter-transference issues. The more a therapist is at ease with themselves and the more they are comfortable with and confident about their competence to deal with any distressing issues disclosed to them, the more likely they will be to establish a safe and trusting base for the survivor.

Guidance through limited re-parenting

I discussed in the first section of this chapter the importance of guiding survivors towards the resolution of sexual abuse and its many negative consequences. This undertaking, or journey as I like to call it, can indeed be treacherous because the survivor may need to tread in uncharted terrain. I have become aware over the years of the immense responsibility implied in this role and the importance of being vigilant to a particular survivor's needs and the aspects of their childhood that were lacking, or that were excessive, and the fact that they will need to be "revisited". While in many instances sexual abuse can occur within what can be termed a perfectly ordinary and, in terms of it being similar to any other average environment, "normal" environment, survivors will frequently recount, in addition to the sexual abuse, other negative or unhelpful experiences.

In some such instances, survivors disclose that their experience of sexual abuse was accompanied by neglect and lack of emotional nurturing by one or both parents or carers, and even siblings. Indeed, in some instances, alcoholism, domestic violence, and physical neglect were also present, as well as inadequate parental guidance in the areas of education, recreational goals, social competence, sex education, and personal effectiveness. On the other hand, survivors have, at times, been subjected to excessive discipline and/or overprotection, or may have had unrealistic or unrelenting parental expectation foisted upon them. In some other instances, survivors may have had to assume responsibility for younger siblings.

Having experienced sexual abuse on its own raises many issues about the personal and social difficulties a survivor is facing, including lack of self-esteem, feelings of self-blame and shame, choosing inappropriate partners, lack of self-efficacy (objective or perceived), difficulty with acknowledging personal needs and having them met, and sexual difficulties. These are some of the effects I have observed as being predominant consequences of sexual abuse, although there are others as discussed in more detail in Chapter 5. The point, however, I wish to make here is that while these difficulties are particularly intense for the individual in any case, they are particularly complex if there have been negative aspects in childhood in addition to the sexual abuse.

I consider that one of my responsibilities as therapist is to provide the opportunity for working through these difficulties within a "limited re-parenting" role, in addition to collaborating with the survivor during the course of their therapy. This relational paradigm was discussed in the previous chapter and it will be "observed in action" in Part III of the book. Suffice it to say that, within such a role and depending on the needs of a particular survivor, I may incorporate aspects of education, personal boundary setting, appropriate praise and reinforcement or explanation about the significance of certain unhelpful acts or behaviours, and guidance when it is necessary or if it is asked for. I have found that the role of limited parent is particularly effective and useful with the younger survivors of sexual abuse, and it is true (as I will be discussing later) that not all survivors require the same degree of guidance or, indeed, lengthy therapy.

The role of limited parent provides the opportunity of experiencing in a limited but, nevertheless, effective manner the process of laying down a solid foundation on which to build self-knowledge, efficacy, and ultimately independence. Ideally, we should all be given the opportunity as children to acquire such a foundation, but the reality is that, even when we have not experienced significant neglect or sexual abuse, we can identify areas where the ideal has fallen short of expectation.

The process of projecting positive and/or negative attributes on to the therapist is one that I find has significance within the role of limited re-parenting. I tend to use reflective observations based on these concepts as illustrative examples when a particular relationship dynamic needs to be addressed. Such an example refers to a situation whereby a survivor may be resistive to collaborating with a particular task assignment, and one possible reason for this may be that she perceives me to be too demanding or insensitive to her needs, as perhaps her father used to be. Making such an observation can trigger very important or relevant discussion that can facilitate emotional processing, especially if guided imagery is also incorporated, and this reinstates the therapeutic collaboration. In this sense I employ the process of projection as a helpful and overt tool, in a somewhat different sense to the implications it has for psychoanalytic therapy. Further examples as well as illustrative discussions on guided imagery are presented in Chapters 9 and 10.

In concluding this section, I should point out that the issue of "power dynamics" in the therapeutic relationship is very important because the experience of having been abused implies that the survivor was subjected to the needs and behaviours of the perpetrator who held all the power, both psychologically as well as physically. Being vigilant about this issue in terms of how a survivor perceives the therapeutic alliance is crucial to the process of engagement and the progress of therapy. Inevitably, either objectively or subjectively, a survivor may perceive the therapist as holding more power than herself. This situation, when coupled with her own feelings of defectiveness, powerlessness, and apprehension, may lead to setbacks, stumbling blocks, or abandonment of therapy altogether. It is important, therefore, to address these potential difficulties as they arise by making use of transference as well as counter-transference as explained earlier.

The final point I should like to make here acts as a signpost to the next section, which concludes the discussion of what I perceive to be my role and responsibilities when seeing survivors of sexual abuse. Although I have alerted the reader to some of the dynamics and processes present in the therapeutic relationship, when looking at the issue of power in particular, I have observed that even though feelings of powerlessness are very strong in some areas, the survivors nevertheless have generally impressed me with their capability and effectiveness in other areas. For example, although one survivor may not be able to make informed choices about the types of relationships that are more suited and rewarding to her on the one hand, she may on the other hand be a very capable student or career woman and very effective at organising her finances. In reviewing the literature about survivors of sexual abuse, I have seldom come across observations that accord these women the credit they deserve. I believe, therefore, that my responsibility as "guide" is to help survivors recognise and acknowledge the areas in which they have competence, strength, and autonomy. In the next section I take up this final point and discuss it within the context of personal growth and independence.

Autonomy through personal growth

The third area of responsibility I believe I have towards my patients is that of leading them towards personal independence and growth. Once again, the adoption of this responsibility has become established and strengthened over the years through the very satisfying observation that individuals are not only able to resolve past abuses, manipulate their cognitive world and accompanying behaviours, and achieve a good degree of emotional literacy, but also they can transcend the requirements of therapy in a self-actualising manner, which we term "personal growth".

I concluded the previous section by mentioning that it is important to acknowledge that most survivors exhibit the ability to have control as well as success in certain areas of their lives and, therefore, they are not totally devoid of power. Clearly, in some instances, the long-term effects of sexual abuse can have negative consequences in most areas of personal as well as social well-being and adjustment, but I would argue that these conse-quences need to be assessed in terms of the whole of childhood experiences and circumstances, as well as the individual's personal and psychological make-up and resources. Although I recognise that the next point I will make may be viewed as controversial, I would like to tentatively propose that survivors of sexual abuse, as well as most people who attend for psychological treatment or counselling (in the absence of serious psychiatric pathology), are able to make consumer choices regarding the level of costs and benefits they are faced with when embarking on treatment. I am reminded here of the words of Abraham Maslow who as early as 1957 remarked that, "Neurotics are not emotionally sick—they are cognitively *wrong*" (Maslow, 1957, p. 129). Most people, however, will be more familiar with Maslow's theories about self-actualisation, and his proposi-tion that all human needs can be arranged in a hierarchy, starting with physical needs, followed by four levels of psychological needs (safety, love, esteem, and self-actualisation).

Maslow further argues that the need to self-actualise is as integral a part of human nature as are physical needs (Maslow, 1957). This becomes evident in the consulting room when a woman who sought therapy has been helped to "right" her cognitions, and make emotional connections: in many instances, she is also able to recognise that the therapy has been an initial step towards greater autonomy and further self-development. I have frequently heard women say, "I never thought I would be able to overcome the past, let alone have so much control over my life. I know I have achieved a lot and can finally experience peace, and although I know this must sound strange, I feel as though there is an anticlimax. Now I feel free to do what I like but I am not sure where to begin. All I know is that there is more to explore".

These feelings are usually expressed towards the conclusion of therapy and are not related to separation anxiety or further unresolved issues. I have now come to recognise them as an expression of a wish for personal growth which lies beyond the issues for which a survivor sought help. I would like to add to this that although these comments are usually made some time after commencing therapy, my own personal view is that "growth" begins the moment a person takes charge of their situation by seeking help. It is also my view that the developmental aspect of growth has no specific beginning or end as such, but is potentially an ongoing state. My role, therefore, as "guide" is inherent throughout the therapeutic process.

This situation is very challenging to a therapist but, equally, it can be very rewarding: I myself have been greatly enriched by some of my clients' strength, imagination, and their journey towards personal growth. It would be true to say that not all people, whether they are receiving therapy or not, will reach such a stage during the course of their lives, although I would like to reinforce the argument that growth is a development concept within a continuum along which all of us hold a place at any point in time. Using this concept, if a survivor wishes to develop further along the continuum, then I would see my role as facilitator of this process, bearing in mind, of course, that I make no judgements and do not hold preset criteria. When survivors are, relatively, at the beginning of their journey towards self-actualisation, I consider that I owe them the opportunity of maximising the potential of their undertaking and in so doing I believe that the following areas are particularly relevant: creativity; flexibility; humour; humility; and self-knowledge. These five aspects are not only required from the therapist for the process of growth, but are also invaluable throughout the therapy and may, indeed, sew the seeds for further development.

I greatly value creativity and my own improvement in this area is a direct result of my work with survivors of sexual abuse, for which I am greatly indebted to them. During the course of my own development and openness to learning and improving not only my interventions but also my inter-personal skills, I discovered the importance of improvising and "creating" within sessions, almost as though I was an artist with a brush and paint pallet. Doing this, however, requires a foundation that is built on sound therapeutic models, extensive clinical experience, and of course self-confidence, because otherwise a little "flutter" into this or that approach may in fact do more harm than good. I also make use of analogies and metaphors when they seem to be appropriate in certain situations and when I consider that they will inspire a particular person. These I might use at any point during the course of treatment. For example, if a patient appears to be particularly stuck and unable to progress, I may use the metaphor that when climbing a mountain it is alright to take a rest along the way at base camp, but that great satisfaction can be gained from completing the journey in spite of the bad weather and fatigue. I find that this theme is a particularly inspirational one because it succeeds in giving permission to slow the progress of therapy or to have setbacks, while creating the necessary impetus to continue.

Flexibility is a good accompaniment to creativity and refers to the importance of being at ease with adjusting certain therapeutic interventions to suit the needs and personality of the survivor. Too rigid an adherence to a particular model and/or its sequential process, may undermine treatment potential as well as impoverish the possibility for further growth and autonomy.

A third element I have found to be excellent is the use of humour (as well as observing it in action) in order to judge a survivor's degree of "freedom from the past". My experience is that, during the early stages of their therapy, most survivors fall into one of three categories with respect to humour. Either they are unable to express or enjoy any humour, or they use humour as a deflection tactic, or they may use it in a sarcastic manner that conveys their anger and bitterness at what happened to them. I have found it very rewarding to observe changes that occur in this area, which often begin in very subtle ways. I am certainly always careful never to introduce humour too early, as this could be interpreted as undermining their situation. The reason I mention humour in relation to personal growth is that in some very delicate way it manages to communicate the degree of autonomy, light-heartedness, and sense of personal comfort a person has reached. A very common example here is when survivors say, "If you had told me at the beginning that my experiences would end up making me a much better and wiser person, I would have shouted at you and would probably never have come back. Now I know that this is the case I can smile to myself and feel a great achievement". This example is certainly not the belly laugh kind of humour, but I consider it to be the kind of "wise humour" that is appreciated once one is in a position of freedom to identify a particular irony or complexity of life. The quote usually leads to a long discussion about the manner in which the resolution of childhood abuse has promoted greater self-knowledge and autonomy.

I will conclude this section by explaining the importance of a therapist's own self-knowledge and humility in their role as "guiding" agents when seeing survivors of childhood abuse. I have already described the variable relating to congruence or genuineness, which I consider to be one feature of self-knowledge. I have also discussed the importance of having an understanding about our own position and attitudes towards those behaviours we deem to be criminal, immoral, unethical, and so on. More specifically, I explained why therapists must have resolved their own personal histories, whether including abuse or not, particularly in relation to their own sexuality. I wish to extend this discussion by including the concept of humility in the constellation of self-knowledge: this was brought to my attention in the course of my work as psychologist, and particularly in my role as therapist and guide. I very quickly discovered that unless I was prepared to have an open mind and accept that not all I had read, been trained in, or encountered during the course of my work was adequate in helping me to be effective with these women, then I would be failing to do my duty by being too rigid and neglecting to observe the most important empirical rule of careful and critical observation.

In this sense I was put, willingly, in a position of humility, whereby, although I knew enough with which to offer the safety, trust, and expertise to help survivors, I nevertheless remained, and still am, very open to learning more and to accepting my limitations. In a sense this is not surprising because the literature on sexual abuse has only gained momentum in the past ten years. I, therefore, feel a great sense of gratitude in having been able and allowed to "journey" with the women I have seen over the past decade. Using the analogy I referred to earlier about the mountain climb, I could say that although I had confidence that I could lead safely, because I knew which path to take, I was not aware of the whole topography. I was also reminded that there is always more than one path available and more than one summit to reach, if indeed that is the goal or personal choice. In this sense, my role as guide towards empowerment, autonomy, and greater self-knowledge is not only to remain vigilant to individual differences, but also the fact that a great deal of my own knowledge and development as guide was the result of being mindful and respectful of these differences.

Conclusions

In the final part of the section on the therapist's requirements I discussed what I perceive my role and responsibilities to be when seeing female survivors of sexual abuse. I defined this role within a framework of providing safety, guidance, and autonomy, which I see as being the essential implications of my responsibilities as therapist. Each aspect of this framework was defined, and then discussed with reference to specific features and also clinical examples.

Finally, there are two observations I wish to make. First, the reader was referred to some of the literature relating to the therapist's characteristics and role. I would like to stress that in my own experience as therapist the variables that I have discussed were not adopted in a priori fashion, but rather they developed and were organised in the manner I described, as a result of my clinical experience with survivors. I, therefore, would like to thank the survivors for contributing to my own understanding and growth. Secondly, the discussion of the framework of my role as therapist within three stages has served as an introduction to Part III, in which I present detailed clinical examples using a three-stage working model.

Part III

The survivors' journey to recovery

Chapter 8

The recovery of survivors: Application of a three-stage working model

INTRODUCTION

The preparation of Part III has been the most intensively challenging, as well as satisfying aspect of my work on this book. The reason for this is that I wished to convey the application of my approach as well as the experience of "journeying" with the survivors along the path of their recovery in the most comprehensive and authentic manner possible. This is, indeed, a huge task because both survivor and therapist undertake a contract requiring full honesty and commitment to the journey, with all that this entails. Inevitably, it is a very personal experience that almost resembles a microcosm of life spanning several years and featuring characters and events that have been instrumental in the survivor's life. I have already acknowledged the unorthodoxy of the writing style of this book, and this will be particularly evident in Part III because most books on therapeutic interventions adopt a more distant and objective stance that betrays very little of the writer's interaction with clients, other than in the most rudimentary sense. While I do not for a moment wish to downgrade such a style (after all, I have myself adhered to it in previous writings), I considered that following it in this instance would do great injustice to the richness of the therapeutic experience, but it would also be at odds with the aims of the book, which has sought to stress the impact my work with survivors of sexual abuse has had on me, both as a person and also as a therapist.

The aim of Part III is to take the reader through the therapeutic process of each of the women survivors whose personal accounts were set out at the start of this book. Consequently, the reader should be alerted from the outset that this chapter is not intended to be a manual on how to treat survivors per se, nor is its purpose to provide detailed instruction on how to use the techniques mentioned. The purpose is to describe each survivor's experience in therapy in a manner unencumbered by lengthy technical detail which, in my view, would distract the reader from the experiential depth of each account. It is hoped that Victoria, Rose, and Florence will be

perceived as real and living people who entered the process of psychotherapy with trepidation but with a great willingness to overcome the past
and to enrich their lives. As promised in Chapter 1, however, I have
accorded each of the survivors' personal histories and therapeutic journeys
due space within which to illustrate all of the issues raised regarding child
sexual abuse (CSA), as well as each of their individual experiences in
therapy. Consequently, I have separated the accounts into three separate
chapters in order that the reader may appreciate them individually.

Before commencing this task, however, I will briefly present the therapeutic "working model" I adopt, as this will consolidate and unite the
issues raised in previous chapters, and will also provide the reader with
the necessary framework for the presentations that follow. The model will
be made explicit during the course of each case study presentation.

A THREE-STAGE, INTEGRATED, WORKING MODEL

In the previous two chapters I discussed the importance of having a sound
theoretical model during the process of psychotherapy. Paradoxically, I
also presented my arguments for the adoption of an eclectic relational
paradigm as opposed to a pure relational paradigm, and supported this
argument by explaining that pure relational stances or "ways of being" may
not always serve the client's best interests due to their potentially inflexible
nature. At the same time, I stressed the importance of conveying consistency to the client by adopting the "limited parent" paradigm because it
lends itself to integrating different stances as appropriate for specific
difficulties relating to each client.

A model that I adopt and which, in my opinion, succeeds in encompassing these arguments—i.e. by respecting the need for empiricism, as well
as the needs and individuality of a particular client—is the three-stage,
integrated, working model (Baker, 1999, 2000).

Engagement

The model, illustrated in Figure 8.1, will become explicit in the three case
studies set out in Chapters 9, 10, and 11, but I will nevertheless offer an
introduction to it at this stage. At first glance, the model appears to be simple
and straightforward, and one that may be argued to reflect the non-specific
and general principles of most intervention techniques. I would agree with
this observation but would like to offer certain qualifications. First, following on from my arguments in the previous two chapters about the importance of "engagement" where survivors of sexual abuse are concerned, I
would assert that this stage is a particularly crucial one that may well
determine not only the survivor's "staying power" in the therapy but also the

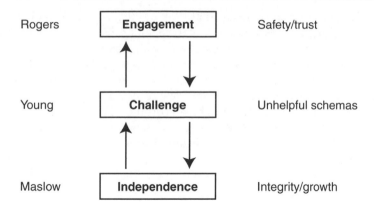

Rogers   **Engagement**   Safety/trust

Young   **Challenge**   Unhelpful schemas

Maslow   **Independence**   Integrity/growth

Figure 8.1   A three-stage (working) model.

outcome on completion. Engagement can be fragile and there is a great need on the part of the therapist to remain vigilant that it is maintained throughout the course of therapy. In my experience, this is not so emphatically the case with clients who have an otherwise adjusted personality and who present for help with very finite and specific difficulties, and where there is no elicited history of childhood abuse (sexual, psychological, or physical). For this group of clients engagement is of course important, but it is my experience that they enter the collaborative process with a completely different set of expectations to those for survivors of childhood abuse. This, I think, can best be explained by the analogy of attempting to sell a product: for the otherwise adjusted individual for whom relationships are not perceived as being problematic and for whom solving a specific problem, such as exam phobia, is the primary reason for their seeking professional help, engagement becomes a function of their confidence in the therapist to provide this service. In this situation, it is my firm belief that I will engage the client if I am successful in "selling" my technique in a manner that is professional, knowledgeable, and of course empathic. In general, such clients are able to accept that they need not like me in order for their therapy to succeed (although this of course helps), and are prepared to collaborate as they would with a driving instructor if they wish to attain their goal. In this sense, it is the respect and trust towards my expertise that I must earn.

This, however, is diametrically opposed to the requirements for engagement where survivors of sexual abuse and also other types of childhood abuse are concerned. In such situations, I have found that the client's engagement with me as a person is not only the primary requirement for a collaborative therapeutic relationship, but it also becomes the perpetual vehicle for consistency and eventual recovery. It is only during the latter stages of therapy when resolution of maladaptive patterns of behaviour and associated emotions progresses that "liking the therapist", or "feeling comfortable" with me assumes a very incidental role. This was very clearly illustrated to me recently, when a survivor who I had seen on one occasion sent me a letter prior to our second meeting because she felt she had to let me know how reassured she was that she "would be able to get on with me", because she experienced me as "easy to be with".

Figure 8.1 emphasises the principles of the client or person-centred approach put forward by Carl Rogers (discussed at length in previous chapters), which has guided me faithfully in this crucial phase of therapy. When the survivor begins to allow me to enter her world through the level of safety and trust I am able to inspire, the second and acutely challenging phase begins to unfold, but there can be no guarantees that engagement will be maintained.

This brings me to the second observation I wish to make concerning the importance of being vigilant to the quality of engagement during the "challenge" phase of the therapy. As will be observed later, the issue of trust is a central feature of many survivors' distress and difficulty in regulating relationships. This "template" of mistrust can be equally applied in "judging" the therapist and there can be no guarantee that just because the survivor engaged in the early part of the therapy she will maintain her level of trust throughout. Collaborating in the challenging part of the therapy, where verbal discourse alone is not enough and when the realisation that translation into action is necessary for change, can activate in survivors the unhelpful patterns for which they are seeking help. A further important complication is the fact that survivors frequently find it very difficult to access their emotions and, therefore, the therapeutic relationship continues to be a primary tool towards change because it provides continuous feedback about how survivors perceive themselves in the therapeutic context, and such information must not escape the therapist's notice.

A final word on engagement at this point is that it may start to be established during the first session (as in the example I offered above) or may take much longer. Each survivor has individual needs in this respect and the important issue to bear in mind is that the "challenge" part of the therapy may not begin without the establishment of a sound collaborative relationship based on safety and trust. This does not simply necessitate that the survivor likes the therapist and feels comfortable with her, but that even when "the going gets tough" and the therapist may not be particularly likeable, she trusts that she will be guided with appropriate care and knowledge.

Challenge

The reason I have termed the second phase of therapy "challenge" is because both the survivor and myself begin to enter uncharted territory.

This is the time when the past is disclosed and its relationship to the present is examined. The reason this is challenging is because it is now addressed in a manner that has the potential to destabilise the survivor's emotional and cognitive status quo. This stage goes beyond the verbalisation and intellectualisation of events and relationship dynamics, although it, of course, encompasses these dimensions. Here, the emotional and cognitive processing or "digesting" of experiences, as I explain it to my clients, begins, and it requires that the survivor is guided towards undertaking certain practical, emotional, and behavioural challenges (which will be made explicit when I present the case studies).

Prior to even attempting cognitive and emotional processing, it is crucial to address a concern very frequently quoted by survivors, and by doing so the term processing becomes understood. Many survivors are perplexed by the fact that they had managed to contain the experience of their abuse in a reasonably satisfactory manner, but then found themselves preoccupied by it to the point of needing to seek professional help. I find that the "deep freeze" metaphor helps in offering an explanation. I suggest the following: events that happen to us as children and for which we have no appropriate mechanism for understanding, may become "stored" or put on ice until such time as we are ready to look at them. At first this fulfils a useful function because it offers us some protection from distress and from being overwhelmed by something we are not able to understand or "digest". Moreover, the effects of early experience can go unnoticed for many years, and even when our relationships with others are affected or when we behave in ways that are damaging to ourselves as well those we care about, we may have little or no insight that what is happening now has a connection with the past. The emergence of survivors' current state of distress is then explained in terms of a two-level cognitive/behavioural therapy (CBT) model that makes use of Aaron Beck's and Jeffrey Young's work (for references see Chapter 6). Beck's CBT is a downward arrow model whereby critical incidents activate basic personal assumptions about the self and the world and these are in turn communicated via negative automatic thoughts that maintain symptoms of depression and anxiety. Returning to the analogy I proposed earlier about the "deep freeze", I attempt to illustrate this process by suggesting that when a critical incident (as proposed by Beck) takes place in a survivor's life—such as losing a loved one through death or separation, becoming a parent, suffering a personal assault, or any life event that has serious implications (which may be negative or even positive)—it can trigger a "power cut" which defrosts what has been hitherto safely conserved. The "flooding" that takes place is the parallel of what Beck terms the activation of beliefs and assumptions, which then precipitates the rise of distress in both cognition and emotion. I explain that the essence of therapy is to start "mopping up" or processing what has been released.

Although not particularly sophisticated, in my experience this illustration succeeds in providing an acceptable explanation of survivors' distress (and even guilt) that they are no longer able to "contain" the events of the past. Indeed, as previously referred to, I find that the use of metaphors can provide very relevant "visual" constructs through which clients can be helped to make sense of their situation when verbalisation may be difficult to access.

While helpful, the above is not sufficient in explaining the survivors' realisation that although they understand the impact childhood events have had on their lives and the process of their re-emergence, they nevertheless almost always express the following: "In a rational and intellectual sense I know what is happening and what I should do, yet I feel powerless to change my behaviour and seem to fall into the same traps". Here, I think Young's SFCBT (schema-focused cognitive behaviour therapy), which I introduced in Chapter 6 and which is a more in-depth extension of Beck's model, succeeds in addressing this next layer or level of the client's distress. Here is where the most pertinent phase of the intervention begins and where the challenge is to first identify and then target the maladaptive schemas or templates that have been established, probably starting from a pre-verbal stage of development. This is challenging because personal maladaptive schemas (PMS) are very enduring patterns with which the individual has learned to make sense of the world, and they are, therefore, very resistive to change. The stubborn and pervasive nature of PMS is that they are regulated not simply by cognitive/behavioural correlates, but also by very potent emotional and sensory variables. Their impact on current experience must, therefore, be subjected to both cognitive discourse (Jehu, 1988; Jehu et al, 1985/6) as well as other "experiential" mediums. The latter is a particularly challenging task as it has the potential to evoke powerful traumatic memories (Smucker et al, 1995), but it is also the one that holds the greatest potential for reversing the widely acknowledged effects of powerlessness, helplessness, mistrust, and guilt resulting not only from the sexual abuse but also from the dysfunctional family dynamics. It should be remembered that both cognitive/behavioural as well as experiential tasks, such as imagery, have been recognised as being necessary adjuncts to the treatment of childhood sexual abuse (Blacke-White and Kline, 1985; Fallon and Coffman, 1991; Resick and Schnicke, 1992; Young, 1994; Arntz and Weertman, 1999).

For the therapist, the challenge is to maintain engagement with the survivor at all stages of the therapeutic journey. The role of "limited parent" is of particular importance, because it provides the means of regulating this engagement even during periods when the "parent" may be perceived as disapproving, punitive, and unrewarding, and most of all confrontational. This process will become evident during the case study presentations, but suffice it to say that this is a task which challenges the resources of both survivor and therapist.

In view of the above discussion, the value of Young's SFCBT model for survivors of sexual abuse, is its rich and acutely intuitive approach, which succeeds in providing a solid theoretical base whilst integrating the wisdom of a number of theoretical approaches ranging from the psychoanalytic to the behavioural.

I should make it clear at this stage that the illustration of the working model I adopt is by no means argued to be special or superior to other approaches. It is one, however, which particularly concords with my personal professional beliefs and orientation, and succeeds in respecting the importance of a sound theoretical base while encompassing the eclectic relational paradigm I have discussed at length. More crucially, however, my ease with this model affords me the professional confidence that inspires most survivors whom I meet with a sense of reassurance and trust that I will be able to guide them with a sufficient level of expertise.

Independence and growth

I have added to the framework so far described a third dimension, which I term independence or growth. These terms may relate to specific and observable gains the individual has made during the course of therapy, but they can also encompass non-specific and personally determined areas of personal growth. In the previous chapter I discussed my role during this stage and explained the importance of acknowledging that for some survivors (as indeed for any individual who enters therapy) there is an expressed need to transcend the requirements of therapy and also the independence gained. To stretch this point further, I made reference to Abraham Maslow's hypothesis that as human beings we have an innate hunger as well as capacity towards personal growth. Maslow discussed the development of this process in terms of personality variables (Maslow, 1957), and I would add to this that in my opinion there exists a state of "preparedness" for that process to take place. What I mean by this is that, while we may all possess such a capacity, not all of us will take advantage of the opportunities that are presented to us at any particular point in time, or ever for that matter. The reasons for this are too complex and, possibly, philosophically based to enter into here, and could constitute a volume in their own right, but suffice it to say for present purposes, I have observed in many of the survivors of sexual abuse a gradual development of this potential and willingness for growth.

What is particularly significant here is to observe the liberation the survivor is experiencing from the perceived "chains" that were previously governing their lives. The picture painted here is certainly not that of Utopia or the unrealistic expectation that the person will never falter and will never again encounter difficulties. Indeed, possibly quite the reverse, in that personal "faults", idiosyncrasies, and the unpredictability of life are now embraced in terms of two realisations—personal responsibility and personal effectiveness. Sigmund Freud's belief that we are not responsible for what we feel and think but must be responsible for what we do, gains particular appreciation here. Moreover, individual pain or suffering is accepted as one of the necessary conditions of life. Indeed, for the more advanced individual (no value judgement is intended here, but simply that personal growth is a very indeterminate journey within which each one of us holds a different place at any one time), pain and suffering are viewed as existential "double-edged" necessities that have the potential of teasing out creative, compassionate, and a host of other instincts, not least that of survival. In this sense, the pain that was triggered by a "critical event" within the context of CBT which I described earlier, and which gave rise to a host of negative psychological symptoms, now becomes the vehicle for personal understanding and freedom towards making informed choices. The reader may recall that I illustrated this progression by quoting a survivor's comment that she was now able to appreciate the gains she had made as a function of her life's experience. I also think that the process of personal growth or the striving for independence is initiated the moment the person undertakes the responsibility of entering therapy, but it is particularly when challenges are undertaken and insight increases that the process gains momentum.

This particular phase of therapy has had, for me, immense rewards. Not only do I have the privilege of having been partly instrumental in allowing these personal qualities to emerge and develop in others, but I have myself been given the opportunity to develop, both spiritually and professionally. It is very difficult to quantify or to elaborate on exactly how I have myself grown as an individual as a result of being a therapist, but I hope that this will unfold during my discussion of the individual case studies. As a professional, it is rather easier to convey the fact that attempting to enter the experience of each individual survivor has stretched to the limit all of the things I have learned during the course of my work and has put me in the position of having to review my working practices. This has, inevitably, benefited the growth of my own insight and expertise and, hopefully, that of the clients I attempt to help.

Finally, I should like to point out that not all of the clients I see follow the progression of therapy I have just discussed. Each individual has different needs as well as different personal resources for dealing with them. One great lesson I have learned is not to brand the client who has opted for dropping out of therapy as a failure. Indeed, I would first ask myself the question: "Have I done everything possible to engage this person?" An additional important issue that has been brought to my attention is that the course of resolving serious childhood difficulties and their consequences does not always follow a linear progression, but is more subject to a developmental progression. In other words, not all clients have the same resources, level of insight, and choice possibilities (whether informed or otherwise) when entering psychological therapy. The reader may recall that I have previously described situations when survivors left therapy, either immediately following the assessment sessions or at other points, and then returned at a later date. This further exemplifies the nature of problem resolution, and more importantly it highlights the importance of the first stage of the working model I have described, which is that of engaging the survivor. In my experience, tackling practical issues in the first instance is crucial as it increases the survivor's sense of empowerment and efficacy, but it also enhances her trust in the therapist as a collaborative and responsible guide, and this of course can only augment engagement potential (Lange et al, 1999; Alpert et al, 2000).

In the Appendix to this book, I have provided a list of recommended reading that includes information on some of the treatment approaches (including guided imagery) I will be referring to in my analysis of the three case histories that follow.

Chapter 9

Victoria

Victoria was referred by her general practitioner. The referral letter was rather brief and stated that she had requested psychological help following her disclosure to him that she had been sexually abused as a child. She had come to the realisation, at the age of twenty-nine, that her personal relationships were suffering as a result of that experience. Her general practitioner was the first person to whom she had disclosed the abuse.

Victoria's completed global rating indicated that her perceived level of functioning with respect to work, home management, and private leisure activities was quite good. Social leisure activities were poor and relationships/communication with others was rated as the worst area of personal functioning. She presented as a very attractive and articulate person. She was very neatly dressed, but in a rather old-fashioned manner, and wore no make-up or jewellery of any sort. There was appropriate eye contact, but she smiled very little and when she first entered the room I detected a strong feeling of discomfort. She sat stiffly on the edge of the chair opposite me and folded her hands on her lap. She said that she felt very awkward and that she had never before been involved in therapy or counselling of any sort. In fact, she said that she was unsure whether she needed help at all and felt guilty about taking my time when I must have "much more needy people to see". She continued by saying that as far as other people were concerned she was a successful and confident young woman who at the age of twenty-nine was holding down a demanding job in the world of finance where she was responsible for managing and training other people. If any of her colleagues were to find out that she was seeking psychological help, they would be shocked because she commanded their admiration and respect for having been successful for her age. In fact, it was not unusual for the younger members of her department to ask for her advice on a variety of issues because they considered her to be level-headed and sensible. The few friends she had would be equally surprised to know she was seeking help, first because she disclosed very little to them about her private life, and secondly because they also viewed her as the "mature" one amongst them who could be relied upon to keep a confidence and offer helpful advice.

When I reflected that she was clearly highly regarded, but could not help wondering who was available to give her this kind of comfort in return, she became tearful and said, "nobody". I went on to say that it must create great pressure for her to be in this position, whereby she is the one who is always in control, to which she replied, "I don't ever remember it being otherwise." Before I was able to respond to this statement, she very quickly followed it by saying that it just occurred to her why she was here and why she was seeking help. She said that about three months previously she had met a man who had come on a business assignment to her firm. They had previously corresponded and talked on the telephone strictly on work-related matters, but they met for the first time when he came over from the mainland. As he was staying for a few days, they had spent a great deal of time together and had socialised over lunches and dinner. She said that for the first time in a very long while she felt some attraction towards this man who was ten years her senior, and said that she had felt comfortable and at ease with him. Her current worry was that following that visit their friendship had developed further and he had visited her on three subsequent weekends, and although some intimacy had taken place, the relationship was not as such consummated. She said that she had strong feelings towards this man and that, although it was still early days, she nevertheless felt that they had a great deal in common and that she sensed that, if she allowed it, the relationship could well be serious and have a long-term future. Her great concern was that she did not know if she would be able to sustain such a relationship because all her previous relationships had ended in "disaster", which she attributed to the fact that there must be "something wrong with me". However, she had now come to the stage that she did not wish to jeopardise her chances in this current situation and felt it was time to seek help.

When I asked her why she thought there was something wrong with her, she looked at me intently and did not respond for some time. For the first time during the session, which was now approaching its close, Victoria's face betrayed some of the pain, bewilderment, grief, and anger she must have been feeling. My instinct was to go to her and hug her and offer her some comfort and reassurance that all would be well, but I felt that this would not be particularly helpful at this stage. I considered that by doing so, her awareness of her emotional vulnerability and need might surface prematurely and I did not wish to disturb the control and equilibrium she had clearly worked so hard towards. I did, however, remain relaxed and non-verbally empathic. Eventually, she said that her GP's referral letter had no doubt mentioned the reason why she was seeking help, which is why she thought there was something wrong with her. She went on to say that she was grateful that I had not referred to this "reason" straight away as she needed time to get to know me and feel comfortable in the situation because she had never spoken to anyone up to now about herself, her feelings, and most of all her past. I responded by saying that it must have taken a great deal of courage, given these feelings, to come to a total stranger and be able to discuss as much as she had already done. I said that she had made a very good start and that I hoped she would come again to continue exploring her feelings and the difficulties she had with forming close relationships. When she asked, "Do you really think I need to . . . will I be wasting your time?" I replied that, her asking me this question conveyed to me further confirmation about her concern towards other people, almost to the point of neglecting her own needs, and that I was able to judge that although she had great strength and ability, she nevertheless had genuine reasons for requesting help. For the first time in the session she smiled and said that daunting as it was for her to allow someone else into her private world, she was grateful that for once someone was able to see below the surface of her controlled and confident exterior. She was also relieved that starting to talk about her life did not inspire the contempt and disapproval she was anticipating, and that although she knew there was a long way to go, she felt that she had managed to take the first step. Before she left, I suggested that it sometimes helps to write things down between sessions, such as impressions following the meeting, any feelings that may have been triggered, or any points that she may wish to discuss at the following session.

FORMULATION

Victoria's situation and her difficulties (as set out below) were formulated following the initial assessment session, six subsequent sessions, and a piece of writing about her life that largely constitutes the account I presented at the opening of Chapter 2. Victoria had experienced the type of childhood characterised by emotional neglect, lack of parental guidance, and sexual abuse by her maternal grandfather. She was the eldest of two children, her younger brother having been born when she was five years old. Victoria's personal description of her early childhood (prior to the sexual abuse) is very significant in that it very clearly illustrates the development of early maladaptive schemas in terms of emotional deprivation and abandonment. The fact that her mother had suffered with post-natal depression following her brother's birth, combined with the constant attention given to him due to his frail health during his early years, created a situation whereby Victoria was spending a great deal of her time alone and was also excluded from building a bond with her brother. In addition, her father's long absences at work, as well as his emotionally distant disposition, was a further significant factor in disturbing the establishment of emotional bonds. The latter was further exacerbated by the loss of various nannies who would be dismissed after Victoria had established an attachment with them.

Left to her own devices for long periods of time, was instrumental in the development of feelings of omnipotence, which, combined with her naturally resilient nature, was initially adaptive in providing the necessary means by which to negotiate a neglectful and disregarding environment towards her personal needs. Her ability to immerse herself in her schoolwork and books, as well as adopting means for dealing with the absence of validation of her by her parents, may have been necessary in her childhood, but in later years this would be the very situation that would prevent her from having the appropriate means to develop close emotional ties. More importantly, the "illusion" of omnipotence in Victoria had clearly developed in her the feeling that only she could be aware of and responsible for her needs, thus giving off the persona that she was a "grounded" and capable woman who no one could suspect of receiving psychological help. Paradoxically, this persona was continually maintaining the situation whereby the love, attention, and guidance that Victoria so much craved was still eluding her.

This situation provides a lucid example of what Freud (1920) termed "repetition compulsion", of which the vehicle for Victoria was the early maladaptive schemas relating to emotional deprivation and abandonment. Although not consciously adopted, they acted as catalysts for her seeking help. In describing her "disastrous" previous relationships, Victoria explained that the men she had been involved with tended to give her mixed messages, whereby they would be available one minute and absent the next. She felt as though she had never quite been "number one" for any of them and would experience great feelings of despair and anxiety when they were not around. Her fear of losing the relationship would make her either withdraw and avoid contact, or become angry and accuse the person involved of having affairs, which would lead to heated arguments and further feelings of abandonment and neglect.

Equally, if she perceived that her partners were cold or unaffectionate, she would swing from becoming demanding and unreasonable to distant and unable to express vulnerability, sadness, or disappointment. Consequently, the relationships would end on a bad note, and this would be irrespective of whether the man was genuinely suitable or unsuitable for her. When the men were exploitative and uncommitted, Victoria would initially be gratified by the generated chemistry, and the perceived feelings of anticipation and longing encompassed in the illusion of "love". However, as soon as the schema of abandonment and emotional deprivation inevitably became activated, she would experience despair at being found once again alone and unloved. On the less frequent occasions when

Victoria's path would cross that of a man who did not, at the outset, generate this chemistry, but who had the potential of holding her in greater esteem and, in time, the potential to be able to fulfil her emotional needs, she would either shun any further contact, believing that the man was "boring" and "uninteresting", or would test the man's resources to such a degree that the relationship would end. Victoria's statement in her personal account—"I do not possess the appropriate mechanism for recognising love when it comes my way"—illustrates this point.

More crucially, the dynamics within her relationships in adult life were particularly disruptive and even destructive due to the added experience of sexual abuse by her maternal grandfather when she was seven years old. At first, her grandfather appeared to provide Victoria with the attention and warmth she needed and this acted as a compensation for the neglect she had been experiencing. The first two years after his arrival in the family household were almost idyllic for her, and he possibly represented for her the first firm memory of a deep bond. This time may be argued to constitute the "grooming" period a paedophile enters into in order to "prepare" for the next stage of boundary crossing between what is appropriate and then inappropriate; it also illustrates Alexander's (1992) suggestion that avoidant or insecure parental attachments are often precursors to sexual abuse (see Chapter 13).

Had Victoria's grandfather not crossed this boundary, the difficulties she was having to face up to may well have been completely different, in that she would have had at least the experience of being loved, attended to, and special, in an appropriately loving manner, and this would have gone a long way towards atoning for the neglect she had experienced at the hands of her parents. The very sudden and brutal experience of fear, incomprehension, and betrayal that followed this idyllic period, at the hands of a figure she had come to love and rely on, was to have significant long-term consequences. Being called "special" by her grandfather, as well as being told that she was his "favourite" while he was abusing her, created in Victoria strong feelings of responsibility and self-blame towards what was happening to her. The feelings of shame and disgust this created, about something she knew was wrong but was unable to comprehend, together with the feeling of having been "cheated", were instrumental in establishing a further maladaptive schema—that of "mistrust/abuse". The latter acted as the primary rubric for monitoring and regulating her relationships, not only with potentially intimate partners but also friendships with colleagues and others. Within this schema, Victoria had internalised a need for remaining vigilant about any potential abuse of trust, even when there was no evidence of objective concern. The latter, coupled with the fact that her parents failed to protect her and stop the abuse, augmented her feelings of omnipotence, in that she believed that only she could take care of herself and that it was too dangerous to let people too close.

In the case of colleagues and friends, the integrity of the mistrust/abuse schema could be maintained relatively easily in that she had the capacity to organise the various aspects of her life in neat compartments that ensured there was no emotional "spillage" from one to another. Intimate relationships, however, represented Victoria's Achilles' heel and became the battleground in which all three schemas were most active and conspired to undermine her efforts to remain detached, safe, and in control of her destiny. With each break-up that followed, the schemas of abandonment, emotional deprivation, and mistrust/abuse would gain further strength and resilience.

In terms of the sexual aspect of her relationships, Victoria did not present with any dysfunction as such, in that she did not experience anorgasmia, dyspareunia, or vaginismus. The level of her sexual desire, however, was very much a function of the quality of the power dynamics within the relationship. Perverse as it may seem to the untrained observer, Victoria's motivation for sex would usually be at its highest during the early stages of a relationship with an ambivalent partner. Her desperate need for emotional connection, and the longing to be validated as a desirable and worthy sexual partner, was driven by the distorted unconscious belief that fulfilling the sexual fantasies and desires of "her man" would ensure this validation and connection. Unfortunately, this situation would be short-lived in that at some point the schema of mistrust/abuse would become activated. Typically, this would happen at the first perceived "sign" of emotional withdrawing or unavailability on the part of the partner (whether justified or not) and she would begin to feel used and abused.

Victoria did not experience particular intrusions in terms of flashbacks or images of the sexual abuse at this point, but the nightmare of the betrayal and distorted dynamics in the relationship between love and sex would become activated. The sexual act for Victoria would assume the powers of an emotional weapon, and possibly the only one she perceived herself to possess. For a time this would appear to bear fruit, but it would simultaneously trigger the start of destructive behavioural patterns within the relationship, and eventually its abrupt end.

The role of Victoria's father in this scenario has not been mentioned so far, and this highlights her own inability to find a place for him in the context of her difficulties. He was barely mentioned in the initial stages of her therapy, and eventually she was able to express a deep sense of grief at having been so distant from him. It could be argued that he represented the first rejection by a male and that this had established the initial doubt in Victoria in terms of her sexual identity and personal worth. This, in addition to the subsequent abuse by her grandfather, constituted a powerful combination in the establishment of maladaptive templates by which to make sense of herself as a woman and also as a sexual partner.

Victoria held far stronger and more ambivalent feelings towards her mother. Her disappointment at the lack of a bond between them, and the apparent lack of concern from her, was far more readily expressed, and her feelings would sway from intense anger to passionate expressions of sadness and loss. Her belief that her mother could have prevented the abuse if only she had taken the trouble to note Victoria's isolation, unhappiness, and the conflicts she was going through as a child, was emphatic. At times, during the "challenging" sessions, Victoria's demeanour would resemble that of a five-year-old who was in need of nurturing, and invited one to assume a protective, "mothering" role, while at other times there would be a shift towards a more distant, suspicious mode. It was during such presentations that the potential for change through guidance via the "limited parent" role assumed its greatest potential.[1]

ENGAGEMENT

Victoria's initial "engagement" process did not present substantial diffi-culties, once her fear of trusting people was addressed and her sexual abuse validated and taken on board. The "critical incident" in the shape of a prospective relationship that signalled to her that it was time to seek pro-fessional help, created the necessary core of current dynamics within which to change unhelpful patterns of behaviour, and in so doing, also to heal the past. Victoria's natural tendency towards logical thinking and problem solving responded well to my explanation of the role of maladaptive schemas in terms of their origin, their resilience, and their destructive potential. The process of therapy was explained, and the point was made that it was collaborative and that we would both be partners in the task aimed at "weakening" the schemas. I explained to Victoria that this process would involve talking as well as "doing" techniques because, without simultaneous behavioural change, emotional distress may not be effectively alleviated.

In particular it was emphasised that there were no "tricks" or covert agendas, because it was felt that this was an important issue to raise given her difficulty in trusting situations that were unfamiliar. However, we did spend some time addressing Victoria's very real anxiety that having kept her life well ordered and protected from the ghosts of the past, it may be in danger of being disrupted by the necessity of disclosing painful material, and the inevitable strength of feeling this would unleash. In response to these fears, I acknowledged that it was expected that some discomfort and pain would ensue, but that at this time in her life she would have the therapy to provide her with the secure base she needed, and I was confident that she possessed the necessary strength and resources to contain her pain. More importantly, I pointed out that people usually monitor how much they are able to face up to at any one time, and that we would adopt a pace she was comfortable with.

CHALLENGES AND PERSONAL GOALS

One of Victoria's initial task assignments was to outline her goals, in no particular order of priority. Her list included the following:

- Come to terms with the sexual abuse.
- Come to terms with her mixed feelings towards her parents.
- Learn to be more relaxed with people.
- Learn to be a little more adventurous, and enjoy life more.
- Understand the reasons why her intimate relationships had not been successful, and most of all, be helped to behave differently and in a more balanced way in her current relationship, which had the potential of being a very special one to her.

The goals were discussed and Victoria's expressed wish was to begin with changing some of her behaviour as regards friends. She also requested some guidance about the general manner in which she conducted her life, which she perceived as being rather "dull, and boring". She said that she wanted to start feeling a little more relaxed and open in her relationships with her female friends, before addressing the sexual abuse in detail. Victoria acknowledged that all the areas she wished to address presented a challenge to her, but that it was possibly the sexual abuse itself and her fear of losing her current relationship that represented the greatest challenge.

I respected Victoria's approach to her therapy, not only because this would provide her with an important initial feeling of confidence that she was dealing with her difficulties in a realistic manner, but it would also respect the premise that this was a collaborative exercise. Consequently, we began by discussing specific areas in which she could start making changes, and here the setting up of "experimental tasks" within a cognitive/behavioural model was worked out between us and the principles of such work was explained. One example of such a task was for Victoria to start recording situations in which she felt she could have behaved in a more open and trusting manner towards her friends. This provided our baseline for cognitive discussion and challenge of what she perceived to be "dangerous areas" and how they could be tested out.

Although risky for her, Victoria engaged well in implementing experiments between sessions, such as starting to talk about her new relationship in more detail than she would have done previously. The result was rewarding to her in that she started to feel a little more "equal' to her friends and also more light-hearted. Following a similar CBT approach, Victoria began to be more outgoing and adventurous towards her hobbies, which had hitherto been of a work-related or intellectual nature. In one particular session she reported that following her enrolment in a fencing class, as well as subscription to a gym, she had started feeling far more relaxed and in tune with her body. She had chosen these particular activities following a discussion of her feelings of inhibition about her body and the fact that she felt more comfortable when conservatively dressed and "well covered up".

The latter observations are typical of women who have experienced sexual abuse, even in the absence of sexual difficulties. For Victoria, as with a great number of survivors, the body is viewed as the source of all their troubles and I have learned that it is important to start by helping them familiarise themselves with their body and "make peace with it" so to speak. Frequently, physical exercise is either fanatically entered into, almost as if the body is being beaten into submission, or at the other extreme it is neglected as though it does not exist. The feedback from women who begin to show appropriate care and nurturing towards their body signals the beginning of increased positive image, as well as integration of mind and body.

SESSION TWELVE

Victoria's sense of self-confidence and ease with herself and with others started visibly growing following the successful completion of a number of other tasks similar to those discussed at the end of the previous section. She came into the room for session twelve, however, looking very unsettled, pale, and almost shaky, and the first thing she said when she sat down was, "Tina, the time has come, I can't pretend with Philip anymore. . . . I think I may have already lost him", and started to cry almost uncontrollably. At this point I went to her and put my arm around her shoulders and we remained in silence for a while.

It is this very crucial moment that I feel as a therapist I must be patient for, as it can signal that the survivor has reached the stage of entering the truly challenging area of therapy. Each survivor enters it at their own pace and, provided certain conditions have been met, then the way is paved for the beginning of schema resolution and "emotional digesting" of key events in the survivor's life. In Victoria's case, the prospect of losing a relationship in which she was starting to invest emotionally in a significant way triggered her abandonment schema, as well as feelings of defectiveness, and I believe that it was her gradual feeling of trust in me as her therapist, which had developed over the preceding weeks, that provided the safe basis on which to start the very challenging work that followed. More importantly, the "safer" and more practical issues we had been working on were positive in instilling in Victoria a sense of growing effectiveness in her personal life and created the necessary confidence in herself and also her therapy.

After she composed herself, Victoria said that when Philip (the man she had grown fond of) had been over from the mainland the previous weekend, the issue of "consummating" their relationship had presented itself and she disclosed to him that she had been sexually abused and was receiving therapy for this. She also told him that she did not yet feel ready to have a full sexual relationship, and although Philip was understanding she felt she had let him down. This triggered feelings in her of anxiety that she would lose him and that he may not be understanding enough to wait.

A few days later she experienced intense feelings of panic and distress and telephoned him to say that she needed a break from their relationship until she had "sorted" her problems out. At this point I said, "Victoria, Philip must be very important to you, and the prospect of losing him hurts. . . . Tell me a little more about how this feels." At this point Victoria's demeanour resembled that of a lost child, who is once again alone and deserted, with her posture virtually closing in on itself as she hugged her body with her arms while leaning forward. She was able to continue talking and said, "This is very difficult for me. . . . No one has ever asked me such profound questions, but I am relieved to be able to show someone how lost I feel. You may not believe it, but for me it is now a matter of life and death. You see, up to now I have always felt that I must either please people to make them love me and accept me, while at the same time I was scared that getting too close would be too dangerous for me. In a way, I've never learned how to behave. . . . Now I want to learn this, because the thought of losing Philip is bringing back terrible feelings of loneliness, and an empty feeling inside which is unbearable. . . . At the same time, it has also become a matter of my own dignity that I do not surrender my body just to keep a man."

I asked her whether these feelings reminded her of how she felt when she was a child. She nodded, and said that since she had told Philip three days ago that she wanted a break from their relationship, she had been unable to concentrate on anything and had waves of feeling physically sick. She said that this is how she used to feel when she was left alone for hours on end, and also how she felt when she had "lost" her grandfather. At this point, Victoria paused in her reflection of the past and silent tears were streaming down her face and she finally looked up towards me in a manner that signalled she anticipated my reaction. My own feeling was that she had a number of needs at this point: she wanted validation for her pain; praise for the connections she had just made; reassurance that I would be able to help; and most of all reassurance that there may be a way out of this extremely painful and testing situation.

I attempted to fulfil these needs by summarising her feelings and by saying that I felt that she was trying to explain that her grandfather had represented the person who had "saved" her from her loneliness, initially, and that she had grown to love him, only to feel betrayed and hurt when he was abusing her, and that she was now feeling that she wanted to be sure that Philip would not exploit her in a similar way. I also said that I felt she was saying that she wanted to make informed choices about when to give herself to a man and that she was right to hold off if the issues were not yet clear to her. Victoria nodded and asked me whether I thought she had done the right thing by telling Philip she needed a break. My response was to ask her what had prompted her to ask for this break. This caused her to reflect for some time and then she said that, when she asked for the break it was done automatically without giving the matter previous consideration, while at the same time feeling that this was the only option open to her.

I volunteered my explanation of this action by suggesting that a number of issues may have been involved. She may have felt that in the absence of a sexual dimension, Philip would devalue the relationship and would leave her. In order to safeguard herself from this repeated pain, she pre-empted what she feared by establishing her own control through the instigation of what she perceived to be inevitable. A further dimension, and possibly one of great importance to her, was that having disclosed to him that she had been sexually abused had activated in her feelings of defectiveness as well as apprehension of what was to follow (i.e. in her therapy), and her schema of mistrust was activated whereby she did not trust that Philip would stand by her, let alone continue to value her after being made aware of such a profound revelation. Her answer to this was, "You have summed it up perfectly . . . please help me sort this mess out . . . whatever it takes. . . . I'm ready to face the ghosts."

Her response was too significant and profoundly valuable to leave unobserved. The reason is that during this session Victoria was, for the first time, actually able to request help in a spontaneously emotional manner, and by so doing she finally acknowledged her vulnerability. It is during such instances that the therapeutic relationship comes into relief and the survivors must be encouraged to express their feelings towards the therapist, and in so doing, confirm the basis of a healthy, nurturing relationship in which the therapist acts as a limited parent. To her statement I replied, "I am so pleased that you feel able to trust me to help you with what has been making you very unhappy for so long . . . how does it feel to be telling me this at this moment?"

Victoria's hitherto very sullen and sad expression showed a flicker of a smile as she looked at me and said, "I never thought I'd be able to say this, but I do believe that you really care, and although I know it's your job to do so, I know I can trust you to see the Victoria I've been hiding away for so long." This comment generated further discussion of our therapeutic relationship and a very crucial issue addressed was the comment that it was "my job to care", and its significance for Victoria. The outcome was that she was able to be reassured that each person I see is "special" in their own individual way, and that being special in terms of being respected and guided in this context is contrasted with being special in an exploitative and abusive manner, as her grandfather had led her to believe.

SEXUAL ABUSE RESOLUTION

Victoria found it difficult initially to verbalise the exact nature of the abuse during the sessions, but she said she would feel safer writing it down in the first instance. Her description of the abuse was discussed very succinctly in the account presented at the start of the book. I have found that survivors must be given time to express and disclose their abuse at their own pace, as the greatest challenge for them is to face up to their deepest feelings of self-loathing, disgust, and perceived responsibility at what happened. In addition, they can never be sure what the therapist's reaction will be and there can be a real concern that the therapist may somehow confirm these perceived attributes. After all, having never spoken in great detail to anyone about this dark secret, how could Victoria envisage what my response would be? Telling me that she had been abused was one thing, but to be explicit about the acts that took place constituted a major challenge for a number of reasons. First, the experience is registered at a time when the child does not possess the emotional, cognitive, and intellectual sophistication of an adult, and it is therefore very difficult to elicit verbally. Secondly, the sheer length of time during which the event has been secretly "nursed" leading up to disclosure inevitably subjects it to a mass of cognitive and emotional distortions whereby misconceptions, self-retribution, and feelings of defectiveness are being reinforced. Victoria's written account of the abuse provided the core material that we addressed over the following sessions. I asked her if she felt comfortable reading it out because in my experience this appears to be the most effective means of processing both feelings and thoughts. Indeed, we stopped several times during the reading as Victoria would become tearful at various points, and this gave us the appropriate clues about which issues were particularly difficult for her. When she finished, Victoria sat very calmly and silent for a while, and then said: "This was the moment I most feared. . . . I was not sure how you would react, but now I've finally done it I feel so relieved. . . . I just wish I had been able to tell my mother."

This was a significant session for Victoria as she began to receive the initial confirmation that she was believed, accepted, and respected despite the horrors of the past. Most of all, she was finally able to verbalise her secret and, by so doing, begin to connect with the emotions that were involved with it. On the other hand, in discussing the account with her, she was able to understand the origins of her schemas and the impact they had on her life, and was also able to start gaining a degree of objectivity. Ironically (as can be the case for many survivors), in reading her account Victoria realised that her grandfather's betrayal, as well as her isolation and disconnection from the family, were by far the most distressing factors, rather than the sexual acts per se. Our work in attempting to deal with these issues involved a number of interventions, the most pertinent being the writing of unsent letters. This is Victoria's letter to her grandfather, which attempts to make sense of her feelings towards him:

> *I don't know what to call you as you stopped being my grandfather the day you changed and started doing all those terrible things to me. . . . But you know, the worst thing is that I loved you so much and I never realised how sad I've been about losing you. Why did you do it? Why did you tell me I was your favourite and then make me feel so horrible and dirty? Why did you betray me and take away the only real love I had as a child? There are so many questions I wish I could ask you, but now you are dead and you will never be able to answer them, let alone apologise for what you did. You know, for years I have been blaming myself and telling myself what a horrible person I must be that I trained myself in the best way I could to hide from the world who I really am! When things go wrong in my relationships and I spend hours crying in my sleep, I can't help thinking that you have destroyed my life.*
>
> *The only thing I have been thankful for is that I am reasonably intelligent and capable and I was able to get away from the house I came to hate, because of all the reminders. Yes, I am successful in my job, and people think I am OK, but this is just a front which hides all the misery inside. I am twenty-nine, and what do I have to show for myself? I have no stable relationship, no children, and don't know how to let go and enjoy myself. I am even afraid to go anywhere new and meet new people because the effort of pretending all over again would be too exhausting.*
>
> *Now I am getting help and, with time, I hope to be able to leave you in the past and start living. I have wasted so much time . . .*

The reading of this "letter" and the debriefing that followed constituted a major breakthrough in Victoria's progress. Not only was she able to link present and past, but most of all she could begin the process of "grieving" for her lost childhood and, in so doing, connect with the corresponding emotions, while experiencing a secure base from which to face up to her "ghosts".

In many instances I find that the reading of material by survivors, which manages to access some of the emotions attached to it, succeeds in dramatically advancing the process of cognitive and emotional "digesting". It is also the case, however, that such an exercise can simultaneously activate the survivor's schemas, and caution must be exercised in terms of choosing the appropriate time within the therapy to carry out such exercises. Moreover, the therapeutic sessions must address the concerns relating to self-blame, responsibility, and damaged self-esteem. In particular, where the issue of who or what is responsible for the abuse is concerned, survivors are very reassured and responsive when I offer direct explanations. Once again, the role of limited parent is crucial towards filling in the gaps of basic educational information and guidance relating to appropriate boundaries between children and adults, while emphasising that responsibility for sexual abuse rests wholly with the abuser.

The discussions that followed the reading of Victoria's material within a schema perspective helped her towards partly fulfilling her initial goals. As a result, she was then able to refine and specify her goals for the remainder of the therapy. These were:

1. To learn how to cope with her feelings of anxiety, fear, and despair when left alone between sessions.
2. To learn practical ways of dealing with "schema activation"— particularly in relationships.
3. To come to terms with her ambivalent feelings towards her parents, and in particular her mother.
4. To learn to like and value herself, and be able to ask for what she needs in her relationships.

Once these goals were defined, the collaborative therapeutic process picked up good momentum and the emotional as well as behavioural aspects of Victoria's personal agenda began to integrate. With respect to her first two goals, Victoria was encouraged and guided towards learning relaxation techniques, while at the same time allowing herself to face up to her anxiety and fear when alone. Most importantly, we discussed the value such feelings can have in terms of deepening the understanding of schema activation, such as abandonment and emotional deprivation, as well as offering the opportunity for her to start the process of nurturing the child within her.

Victoria suggested that she would prefer to refer to her schemas as "buttons", which when pushed activated her feelings of isolation, fear, etc. For schema resolution, Victoria started keeping a diary in which she recorded the triggers that activated her "buttons", and the emotions, thoughts, and behaviours these set off. The diary provided our baseline for discussions in terms of "healthy" versus "unhealthy" reactions, and realistic versus unrealistic concerns. This information also helped Victoria in the construction of flashcards which she found invaluable for coping between sessions. One such flashcard read:

Right now I feel very scared and alone because Philip has not rung me for a while, but I know that the reason I feel this way is because my abandonment button is being pushed and this intensifies the feelings I have had for most of my life. Even though I feel very alone, I know that this has nothing to do with Philip because, after all it was me who suggested we did not see each other for a while. So, although the feelings I have now

are painful, I understand how they've come about, and I could test out my
theory by getting in touch with him myself.

The work relating to nurturing the child within was very crucial in terms
of "self-healing", personal forgiveness, and integration of Victoria's whole
being. Following on from our sessions, she agreed to attempt allocating
special time for this purpose, whereby she would visualise herself as a child,
while being soothed and comforted by her adult self which was stable and
in charge. Victoria appeared to benefit from such experiential tasks,
particularly as we had agreed that she could contact me by telephone at my
office should the need arise.

The negotiation between survivors and myself regarding such contact is
subject to the requirements of any given individual. It is a dimension of the
therapy that must not be taken for granted as it is important to define the
boundaries between pre-arranged sessions and contact outside them. In the
case of Victoria, she was mostly wary of imposing on my time and she
exercised extreme caution about not abusing our arrangements, either by
being late or not attending without explanation. This caution was based on
Victoria's internalised belief that she did not deserve care and attention and
so she must comply with gratitude to the requirements of her therapy.
When I suggested at this very crucial point in the therapy that she could
contact me if she ever felt overwhelmed or in need of support, she thanked
me but maintained that she did not envisage needing to disturb me. I
therefore considered it hugely significant to her progress when on two
occasions she did avail herself of my offer, prompted by very intense
feelings of sadness triggered by her visualisation work. Far from being
negatively overwhelmed, however, Victoria rang me because she said she
wanted to share with me her intense feeling of relief and success in starting
to make peace with the past and, mostly, with herself. In further discussion
about her action at our subsequent session, she said that up to now she had
never felt that she had someone with whom to share important milestones
in a spontaneous manner, and the fact that she had lost her inhibition
about contacting me signalled to her that she had progressed a great deal.
Indeed, this particular discussion paved the way for the resolution of her
ambivalence towards her parents, and in particular her mother, because it
highlighted the absence of parental interest and guidance.

GUIDED IMAGERY WITH RESCRIPTING

For our guided imagery exercise (see the notes to this chapter[2] and also
Chapter 14), Victoria picked an incident when she was twelve years old that
involved her mother. She pictured herself coming from school in particularly jovial mood because her teacher had made a point of complimenting

her in front of the class about a piece of work that she said was excellent. She remembered that all through the journey on the school bus she was feeling elated and could not wait to get home to tell her mother. On arriving at the house her mother was busy with some paperwork and Victoria burst into the room saying she had to tell her what her teacher said about her at school. She remembered that her mother barely looked up from what she was doing and said "no doubt something very good dear . . . your father and I know how hard you work, so it doesn't come as any surprise to us." Victoria described how she felt instantly deflated and was then able to verbalise that what she really craved was for her mother to leave what she was doing, to go to her, and give her a hug.

Victoria became tearful the moment she was able to connect with the fact that it was the affection and warmth she had so craved from her mother. In addition, she realised that her efforts to get this attention were mostly aborted, and was able to connect this with a pattern of trying to win the affection of others. When the latter failed she compensated by strengthening her resolve to strive even harder in the areas she felt she had control over—i.e. her personal achievements—but alas, in her perception the gains were rather hollow.

Following the debriefing of this first stage of the guided imagery exercise, we resumed it in order to exploit its potential for changing the roots of the emotional deprivation schema via role-play. In other words, Victoria "re-entered" the scenario at the point when mother appeared to be dismissive and I role-played the mother's part:

VICTORIA: Mother, I know you appreciate the fact that I do well at school, and I don't wish to complain, but sometimes I so much want to tell you more about what I'm actually doing . . . you never seem to ask questions.
"MOTHER":   Victoria, are you saying that I'm not interested in you?! You must see how busy I've been, and you know I'm not always in the best of health. . . . I can really do without being made to feel guilty. . . . I do my best.
VICTORIA: Mother, I know you do your best and I really worry when you're not well, and please don't feel guilty, I'm just trying to say I miss you sometimes because I love you, and wish we could be closer. [In the imagery, Victoria goes to her mother and hugs her.]
"MOTHER":   [Hugs her back.] I may not always show it, but I do love you . . . very much. You seem to be so grown up, I forget that you need me. . . . I will try not to forget.

Exercises such as this helped Victoria to begin assuming that she could have the means by which to change the course of events in her life, and although they were simply symbolic, they were nevertheless cathartic and very powerful in allowing her to appreciate the complexity of parent/child dynamics. The latter was particularly helped by Victoria role-playing her mother. In relation to the current state of her relationship with her mother, Victoria volunteered to get in touch with her family and also to suggest a visit as she had not seen them for almost a year. She later described the main outcome of the visit as being a feeling of freedom from unrealistic expectations about her parents' behaviour. In other words, she was accepting of the fact that her mother did not appear to have the necessary resources for behaving as the ideal image Victoria held about how a mother should be; equally, she was able to appreciate that her father would most likely remain unable to change into a more emotionally accessible man. Consequently, she opted for not disclosing the abuse to them, but felt that it would be worthwhile attempting to negotiate a different type of relationship with them. In discussing this, she said that while she did not particularly feel the need for excessive contact with her parents, she had reached a stage where she did not feel compelled to avoid them and wished to maintain a reasonable amount of contact. When asked what made her come to this decision she said, "I feel as though for years I must have had a secret wish for my parents to wake up to the fact that I am still a child and need their care and concern. Because I was not getting what I wanted I felt hurt and angry with them and so it was easier to avoid them. Now that I am starting to grow up inside, I realise that I don't need them in the same way . . . but they are still my parents, and in their own way they have done their best. Who knows, one day they might need me, and I want to be there for them."

SESSION TWENTY-EIGHT: REVIEW AND FURTHER PROGRESS

In reviewing Victoria's progress in order to assess her gains and remaining needs, she asserted that she had reached a point whereby "a veil had been removed" from in front of her eyes, and she could see more clearly. She also said that although there was still a degree of sadness about her life, this was different to the despair she had experienced and she was able to start accepting the abuse and her parental neglect. In terms of her remaining needs, she said that she wished to continue building on her self-esteem, and learning to be bolder about asking to have her needs met, when appropriate. She emphasised that she wanted to put her "freedom from the past" to good use and not lose touch with herself now that she was finally able to connect with her emotions.

Interestingly, the issue of Philip, although still very important to her, had lost some of its urgency. Philip had, in fact, written to her saying that he was not putting pressure on her but just wanted to let her know that he was still thinking of her and that he hoped she was progressing well in her therapy. He also said that he was there for her whenever she was ready to talk. When asked about her reaction to the letter, Victoria said: "It is so strange you know . . . when I think that I actually finally got the courage to seek help because I was so scared of losing Philip, and yet now I feel I am finally there, I'm not sure that I am really ready to commit myself". I responded by saying: "When you say, 'finally there', what do you mean?" Victoria replied that although she had entered therapy for her own sake, at the back of her mind she had held on to the idea that when she was "well" she would become a worthy partner for Philip. She went on to say, however, that as she worked through the various stages of her therapy, her greatest gain was to feel emotionally independent and that her sense of worth was entirely an issue for herself and it did not have to be measured against someone else's opinion. Having explained this, she said that she still cared a lot for him but was not sure at this stage whether she wanted to pursue the relationship. She said she had a feeling that there was a lot more to explore first.

CONCLUDING SESSIONS: INDEPENDENCE AND GROWTH

In my opinion, Victoria's remarks signalled the start of the third stage of her therapy. In other words, she was beginning to reap the benefits of her hard work in terms of insight and greater emotional freedom, but she was also beginning to realise, possibly for the first time in her life, that she could make choices that were not governed solely by the cycle of repeated and unhelpful patterns of behaviour. This is an example of what I term "growth", and in the case of Victoria I experienced, as I always do during such stages, an immense sense of joy and anticipation about what she would decide to do next.

Something that I find difficult to describe is the day when a survivor walks into my room and something tells me they have literally turned a corner. It is not merely their words which signal this event, but their whole body posture, general demeanour, and facial expression. One day, a few weeks prior to concluding the therapy, Victoria came to see me looking very different to how I had been used to seeing her. She had changed her hairstyle and had substituted her rather old-fashioned clothes for something much more colourful and fashionable. It was the first time she had actually walked into the room with a smile on her face, and her general presentation was of someone who was remarkably at ease with herself.

I felt I was being invited to comment as she entered, and I said: "Victoria, you look so happy, and also very different. . . . I mean this positively, of course . . ." She replied by saying: "It's very strange, but last week I felt that my life was about to begin and I wanted to celebrate this discovery by being adventurous and doing something different. So I decided to change my image . . . and this is only the start." She went on to say that she had spoken to Philip on the telephone and told him that she hoped he would come over at some point as she felt that she had unfairly pushed him away and wanted to explain things face to face. In this session she said that she had realised that Philip had indeed been a very thoughtful and caring man, but at the same time she also realised that her despair about the prospect of losing him was based on need and the fear of being alone. She took great care to explain that this time she was not pushing him away because he was "nice" and she therefore became bored with him, but rather that she was now "choosing herself" over any relationship. More-over, she said that rather than run away from confrontation as she previously did, she wanted to face him and explain her reasons for bringing their relationship to a close. This was important to her because she wanted to return the respect that he had shown her, but most of all she wanted to take the opportunity of seeing herself addressing her needs in a responsible and adult manner.

Victoria's personal growth in terms of self-esteem and freedom was powerfully expressed in the above account, which paved the way towards the conclusion of the therapy and the start of her new life. Indeed, the remaining sessions became the focus of her future plans and, of course, the end of the therapeutic relationship. Victoria continued to require guidance and feedback about what she was planning and she said that she had come to look upon me as the only mentor she ever had. She also said that although she infrequently availed herself of my help other than in her sessions, she was reassured by the fact that I was there if she needed me. This particular feedback was very valuable in addressing her potential anxieties about "being alone", and she said that this was the reason why she needed to "test" herself before becoming attached to anyone else. The opportunity for such a test presented itself in the shape of a possible transfer from the firm in which she was working to another European country for a period of one year. Her employers were so impressed by her work that they wanted to use her expertise in setting up a similar depart-ment overseas.

The advantages and disadvantages of such a move were discussed, and Victoria said that although she was flattered by this promotion it was the potential challenge of further personal growth that attracted her. She felt that it was time to move away from the relative safety she had structured for herself after completing her education, and she hoped to push herself towards meeting different people and experimenting with different leisure interests. I chose at this point to ask her the following question: "Victoria, using the metaphor of climbing a very high and treacherous mountain to describe your journey through this therapy, where would you place yourself at this point?" Victoria reflected for a while and said, "I am relieved and elated by the fact that I have already covered so much ground and I am now taking a short rest about 1,000 feet from the summit. It is sunny, and while I'm gazing over the distance I have travelled, I can see clearly all the way to the foothills and feel amazed that I have come so far. Above me lie further challenges, but I feel that I have become fitter through the climb and know I can continue on my own. . . . Although no doubt I will need further short breaks, I can't wait to feel the fresh breeze at the top, and see the panoramic scenery, and know that I've almost conquered the mountain!"

This was a truly profound and very emotional moment for both of us. The instant Victoria realised what she had just said, we looked at each other in silence, and the growth elements of her very personal "journey" were crystallised. These elements can be explained as follows:

1. The therapy had reached a stage whereby there was a deep understanding between us that transcended the need for words. This exemplifies a particular aspect of growth when events need no longer be exhaustively explained, as the richness of the insight gained lies not in words but in the depth of intuitive perception.
2. An additional growth element in Victoria was displayed in the fact that for the first time during the therapy she became aware of me as a separate person, and not only as her therapist, mother, or mentor. I was made aware that she needed to show her empathy towards my own elation at her words by coming over to give me a hug.
3. Victoria's description of her remaining mountain trek implied that for the first time she was approaching life with autonomy, confidence in her resources, but most of all curiosity about what lies ahead. It is my belief that it is only when we are truly integrated and self-accepting that we become able to be genuinely curious about life and others, and Victoria was just beginning to enter this experience.

FINAL COMMENTS

Victoria belongs to a group of survivors of CSA who have not suffered substantial personality disruption as a result of their experience. The reasons for this can only be speculative and may involve a host of individual, environmental, and biological factors. Suffice it to say that her story presents a good illustration of survivors who are able to maintain stability in certain areas of their life, particularly those that can be relegated to compartments that do not compromise the survivor's emotional integrity. It is her personal and intimate relationships that presented Victoria with her biggest and most painful challenge, and the long-term sequelae of her sexual abuse, therefore, may be said to best conform to the developmental model (Cole and Putnam, 1992; Alexander, 1992) discussed in Chapter 5. Issues succinctly illustrated in Victoria's story related to the quality of parental attachment, identity confusion, self-criticism, and, most importantly, the social problems she encountered in terms of isolation, distrust, and insecurity in relationships.

The schema-focused approach was especially relevant in helping Victoria to resolve these difficulties, particularly as it incorporates cognitive/ behavioural techniques which, in the early part of therapy, enhance the argued prerequisite of helping the survivor gain competence and self-esteem prior to tackling the sexual abuse (Lange et al, 1999). Indeed, in Victoria's case there was no indication of a need for the implementation of intrusive experiential techniques, such as imagery, for resolving her sexual abuse. Working with the information she volunteered was sufficient in validating her experience and in helping her resolve her feelings of guilt. The imagery involving her mother, however, was cathartic and very pertinent in working through her emotional deprivation schema.

Victoria's presentation can be said to conform to the 18 per cent of survivors whom I have seen, who in terms of absence of psychiatric and impulse control difficulties, or conclusive personality disorder, are outwardly and subjectively perceived to be "coping well", at least in managing the practicalities of daily life. The account that follows is representative of those survivors whose experience of childhood sexual abuse has had a greater impact on their resources for managing daily life. The overall "working" label that encompasses the emotional and functional coping level of the survivor whose progress in therapy is presented in the next chapter, can be said, at presentation, to have been at "bad".

Chapter 10

Rose

BACKGROUND TO THE FIRST SESSION

Rose was thirty-two when she was referred by Relate. She had been advised to seek help from them by her general practitioner after repeated visits to him for complaints of a gynaecological nature, for which a number of investigations were carried out but did not reveal any organic problems. Eventually, Rose plucked up courage and told her GP that she very much wanted to resume her sexual relationship with her husband, which had gradually declined after the birth of their three-year-old daughter, but she simply had no desire for it. Rose did not, however, disclose to her GP that she had been sexually abused as a child, and was promptly advised to seek help from Relate, who provide sexual and marital therapy.

Rose followed this advice, motivated strongly by her wish to please her husband Tony, who was very keen to accompany her. Because the quality of the marital relationship was very good, the Relate counsellor embarked on a straightforward sex therapy programme, unaware of Rose's past, which she had chosen not to disclose. Prior to the couple's fourth session, however, Rose telephoned the counsellor and told her that she did not feel able to continue with the sessions. When prompted to give her reasons, Rose broke down and started crying, saying that she found the tasks too hard to carry out and also that she felt guilty because her husband had been very patient and understanding, but he did not know how Rose felt. The Relate counsellor was experienced and sensitive enough to suggest that Rose would be welcome to see her by herself to discuss what was troubling her, if she felt this would help. Rose took up her offer and when she saw her said that each time she was about to start the prescribed exercises she would get very disturbing flashbacks about her past. This was the first time Rose had remotely mentioned her abuse, and she responded to gentle probing by finally disclosing the fact that her father had abused her between the ages of nine and fifteen years. She did not disclose any further details at that point, but a number of other issues about her life that Rose volunteered alerted the counsellor to the fact that Rose's difficulties fell outside the domain of her expertise and suggested a referral to a clinical psychologist.

This chain of events was to bring Rose to me for therapy at a time when she had sunk to a very low point in her life. The positive outcome of her session with the Relate counsellor was that the latter's sensitive and thoughtful handling gave rise the beginnings of hope that she was not a freak, but most of all it gave her the courage to finally disclose her past to her husband.

FIRST SESSION

Rose cancelled a number of her first appointments, usually saying that the times were not convenient or that she had no babysitter. The first time she entered my room I had to consult my notes for her date of birth because she looked much younger than her thirty-two years. She was quite slight in build, had very short blonde hair framing a very pretty face that was subtly made up, and was neatly dressed in a black trouser suit. There was a definite sense of edginess as she sat down and she looked directly at me in a rather challenging manner that I found quite unnerving. It was as though her expression was saying, "You may ask me what you like, but I won't tell you!", or "I don't know what I'm doing here because you can't help me."

I started off by saying that I was pleased to meet her at last. She did not reply and so I went on to say that the referral letter had explained why she was here and I summarised this to her. At this point, she lowered her head and said, "I know I should be grateful to the very nice lady I spoke to at Relate as it was the first time I was able to tell anyone of my nightmare, but to be honest, I'm not sure whether I want to continue with this". When I asked her to explain what she meant by, "this", she said that it was all very well in this day and age for people to want to "spill out their guts" to "do-gooders" and "listening/caring people", but that she doubted that in her case this would do *her* any good. I responded to this by asking her why it was that she had not cancelled her appointment with me altogether, since after all it was her choice whether she wished to see me. She was quiet for some time, not making eye contact with me, and then said that she was torn between wanting to make things "better" for her family and not wanting to go through the "whole bloody business again". I responded by saying that she seemed to be in a very difficult situation indeed, as clearly she must love her family very much to be finding herself in such a dilemma, but I wanted her to help me understand how coming to see me would help her make things better for her family?

I was able to sense that Rose found this question very challenging and she was on the verge of tears, but she exerted control and was clearly making huge efforts not to let me see the extent of her distress. She was continually rubbing her hands. My attention was directed at these hands, which, small as they were, expressed so much. Not only did they convey the discomfort and anxiety Rose was feeling, but they also had a curious angry appearance, both in they way they moved and also in the way they looked. The nails were very short and uniformly cut, almost too close to the cuticle, while the colour of the skin on the hands was a strong pink against a generally pale complexion, suggesting she either did a lot of hand washing or had some dermatological problem.

Eventually, Rose replied to my question by saying: "For many years I did things my way and did not give much thought as to whether they were 'normal of not' . . . now I have my own family, I can't help feeling that there is something very wrong in some of the things I do. . . . I love my husband and daughter too much to let them suffer because of me." I was acutely aware that Rose was clearly finding it very difficult to come to the point about what was troubling her, but I felt that unless I managed to break through some of the ice she would not return. I reflected for a moment and then said, "Rose, I can't help feeling that you being here is causing you a lot of grief and discomfort. . . . You are right, why should you have to tell me very personal things, when you have no idea whether I will understand, let alone be able to help you. . . . At the same time, I also can't help feeling that you love your family so much that you were prepared to come here and put up with your discomfort . . . so let's try between us to see how we can help the situation."

For the first time in this session, the tension on Rose's face eased up slightly and the angry, diffident look softened. She said rather quickly and in rushed sentences: "I clean too much, worry too much, and hate sex. . . . It won't be too long before my daughter notices that her mum is not normal." She dropped her gaze and then looked up at me, probably to read my reaction. By now I was sensitised to the fact that everything I said or did could have far-reaching effects, either one way or the other, and so I remained very calm and looked at her in a manner not dissimilar to that of a mother who feels for her daughter's discomfort and wants to convey to her that she loves her all the same and is proud of all the efforts she makes. This is the type of non-verbal, empathic posture that can create an important shift during a very precarious moment in the engagement process. I was, therefore, relieved when even before I was about to respond to her disclosure, she continued by saying, "You see, my mother was not normal. . . . For a start, I don't even think she loved us, as children. But it's not just that. . . . When I left home to get away and worked as a nanny, it was a shock to me to see how other mothers behaved. I would be destroyed if my own daughter felt about me as I now feel about my mother."

I felt sufficiently emboldened to ask how was her mother different to those other mothers she had met. It seemed vital not to allow the momentum of her disclosure to falter. She seemed almost relieved by my question and nodded in an absent-minded manner a few times before responding, "I feel I'm being disloyal by saying this, but I think there must have been something seriously wrong with her. She must have definitely hated sex too because she always used such angry, foul language when talking about anything remotely related to sex. I used to wonder how we had actually come to be born. . . . In the households where I've worked since leaving home, the women talked about sex in a free manner, and they were able to actually smile, or even make funny jokes about it. They were also not constantly uptight like my mother used to be, and were not obsessive about cleanliness and constantly doing housework."

There was a great deal of material to respond to, but I felt that the most important aspects here were to acknowledge Rose's confusion about her observation of apparent differences in "mothers"; her concern about not wishing to damage her family by depriving her husband and transmitting unhealthy attitudes to her daughter; her distress about realising she had a less than "ideal" mother; and, most of all, reward her for showing courage by being able to start addressing very important and personal issues. With respect to the sexual abuse by her father, I was sufficiently alerted to the fact that Rose had no intention of even alluding to it during this session, and I respected this. When I finished making my observations we were nearing the end of the session and Rose said that although it was difficult to start talking about her life, she felt it would be worth continuing for a while to see if I would be able to help her. I realised that in putting it this way, she was allowing herself a "way out" should things get too difficult for her and she was, therefore, warning me. In order to create a link between this and our subsequent session, I considered that it would be important to reassure her that I understood what she was saying, and, in addition, impart in some small but effective manner the process of collaboration and feeling of effectiveness (on both parts) by targeting practical issues. To that end, I explained the basic principles of cognitive/behaviour therapy and that we would both be partners in trying to work through the problems Rose chose to bring to the sessions. I also stressed that she would be the one to decide which problems she wished to start with, and suggested she might like to create a list of the issues she wished to address with me, and that she could order them in terms of their "difficulty".

After we arranged the next appointment and Rose was about to leave, she hesitated for a moment and then just before getting up she said, "Oh, and I forgot to tell you one other thing. . . . I'm sure it's not normal to want to hurt yourself, but this is what I used to do in the past . . . all over my arms and legs. . . . I'm terrified that I will start to do this again . . . how will I hide it from them?" These "last minute" reflections are not infrequent in my experience and must be handled with great care. A balance must be created from the outset regarding, on the one hand, the observation of appropriate boundaries, and on the other an understanding of the reasons something is being said and its importance for the survivor.

In closing our session, I responded to Rose's question by saying: "Rose, you've just told me something very important and I am very pleased that you have done so . . . it means that you are beginning to trust me. Although we have no time to discuss this further, I want you to know that I have taken on board what you've just said and we will continue to talk about it, if you wish, at our next session. In the meantime, it may help if you could keep a record of each time you feel you may want to hurt yourself; this will help us to understand how best to deal with the problem." Rose nodded, shook my hand, and left.

INITIAL FORMULATION

Rose cancelled two further appointments following her initial session with me. It was six weeks before I saw her again, and this allowed me time to go over the events of our first meeting and start formulating the problems (at this stage I had no details of the sexual abuse, other than the fact that the perpetrator was her father). Rose, aged thirty-two years; presented initially in a very tense and angry manner. She was clearly conflicted between wishing to create a loving and stable home for her family, while having sufficient insight to realise that she had been damaged in some way as a result of the sexual abuse and also her mother's attitudes, behaviours, and general demeanour towards her. She appeared to hold great resentment about having to talk about herself, which would, in her perception, put her in a vulnerable situation that held unknown "dangers". My initial observations of Rose were that she had a great need for control; I also suspected that there existed a compulsive element to her personality based on her parting comments about self-harm and my "hunch" that she engaged in obsessive behaviour—note my observation of her hands, her mother's compulsive cleaning, and Rose's fear that she was like her); intense lack of trust and extreme difficulty in negotiating a working relationship; avoidant behaviour; and sexual difficulties characterised by intense revulsion. In psychiatric terms Rose could be said to present with a "mixed personality disorder", with traits of borderline, obsessive compulsive, and avoidant personality disorders (DSM III-R, American Psychiatric Association, 1987).

I had not elicited sufficient symptoms to justify a diagnosis of clinical depression at that stage, although I suspected a moderate degree of anxiety. I discussed the role of personality disorder in survivors of sexual abuse in Chapter 5, and must now clarify that in my clinical work such diagnoses serve only as a general guide that aids the identification of unhelpful personal schemas. In Rose's case, this initial formulation alerted me to the fact that, for her, unrelenting standards, subjugation, defectiveness, social exclusion, and of course emotional deprivation, would all be central to our work. More importantly, I was sufficiently alerted to the fact that for Rose, the dynamics within our therapeutic relationship would require particular and careful attention and that gentle confrontation would play an important role. This realisation also alerted me to the fact that the engagement process would not be an easy one and that I would have to be particularly vigilant at our next session to ensure that Rose would remain in therapy.

Rose's global rating form indicated that she subjectively considered she had moderate to severe difficulties in most areas of daily living, namely, social and private leisure activities; home management; and relationships with others in terms of communication, and with her husband in terms of sexual behaviour. My overall initial impression was that Rose was coping badly at the time she presented for therapy (for coping level categories, see Chapter 4).

ENGAGEMENT: SECOND SESSION

Rose apologised for cancelling her previous two appointments, saying that the times proved to be inconvenient after all. Given the above observations I considered it would be important to address the issue straight away and I said, "Rose, I appreciate that it must be difficult for you to find time to come here, but it is important that we discuss these difficulties and make sure you allow time for yourself. . . . When I thought about the things we discussed at our last meeting, I realised that you were right to come along and that it is important that we have regular sessions." Rose was taken aback by my approach and she looked at me with a mixture of anger and relief. She had clearly not expected me to confront her and said, "It sounds as if you're telling me off. . . . I didn't think you'd even notice that I cancelled my appointments, after all you must see so many people. . . . The truth is, I always have so much to do and it's not easy finding babysitters. Also . . ., after I blurted out at the last minute last time about my hurting myself, I wasn't sure what you would think of me. . . . I've never told anyone about it."

There were clearly a host of issues to be addressed in Rose's response and this constituted a large part of our session. This took place specifically in terms of our therapeutic relationship and focused on her feelings that she was just "one of many patients" and, therefore, unimportant; her tendency to put others first and not finding time for herself; the need to observe certain boundaries in our work and explanation of my limited parenting role; her anxiety about needing my approval; and of course the self-harm issue. Indeed the latter signalled the first targeted area for cognitive/behavioural intervention.

Predictably, Rose had not completed a list of goals, nor had she kept a diary, but during this session the engagement process truly began as Rose's perception of me and the therapeutic situation began to inspire her with confidence that her concerns were being addressed. It confirmed to me once more the need to be supremely vigilant about the interaction in the here and now by not allowing important material to slip through. This is not to say that Rose's engagement remained constant from there on, but we managed to reach an important contractual understanding that honesty would be paramount and that when this was difficult to maintain we would discuss the reasons why.

During this session we discussed response prevention techniques in relation to the self-harm, and rehearsed practical techniques with which to tackle feelings of tension and frustration. I reinforced the importance of keeping a diary of events in order that we could begin to make connections. I also explained the value of listing her goals in terms of their current relevance to her life. Rose assured me she would do this and apologised for having been "difficult". However, the most important aspect of this session which truly "broke the ice" was when she said, just before ending our session, "I'm so grateful to you for not wanting to know about the abuse straight away. I realise now how afraid I've been about having to actually talk about it. But I have a feeling you must know that most of my troubles stem from this disgusting business. . . . I've been trying to kid myself that I could just put it behind me. . . . For the sake of my family, I will try my best to do what it takes to chase away those horrible ghosts."

EXTENDED FORMULATION AND THERAPY PLAN

With the benefit of ten further sessions, Rose's diaries, and her personal account (see Chapter 2), I was able to complete my formulation. Rose's personal account was part of a structured approach towards cognitive and emotional processing, which requires that the survivor writes several statements of the actual sexually traumatic event. This is a well documented approach that is particularly effective for survivors of rape (see Resick and Schnicke, 1993).

Rose's family background was one in which religion played a big part and where her mother was the authoritarian figure for whom the Catholic religion acted as a shroud for her own unresolved conflicts with sex, personal identity, and extreme anxiety about losing control. From a very early age, Rose began to fear her mother and was never able to develop a bond with her. She had a close relationship with her siblings, but her eldest brother was six years her senior and he very quickly began to rebel and spent very little time at home. Her mother's progressing difficulties in regulating her environment due to obsessive compulsive behaviour in terms of constant cleaning and checking, eventually led her to start "losing her grip", and her verbal abuse and angry temper escalated. Rose became very protective of her younger sister and would try to appease her mother and would willingly put herself in the firing line of her mother's tempers in order to shield her sister.

By the age of nine she was a little girl who was already beginning to shoulder a great deal of responsibility, and her own individual needs and her personal identity were never responded to or allowed to flourish. Indeed, it could be argued that Rose played a very important part in maintaining the "apparent" (dysfunctional) stability in the family in her role as protector towards her sister, and sex object for her father's gratification, thus absolving her mother from her "sexual duties". Her father was a passive figure who did anything for "a quiet life". Rose had been fond of him but in retrospect realised that he had never done anything significant to protect his children from their mother's verbal abuse.

Her world was completely shattered the day her father effectively raped her; this, coupled with the fact that, not only were her mother's maternal and protective instincts severely lacking, but were positively geared towards cruelty, neglect, and (arguably) collusion with sexual abuse, had a serious impact on Rose's childhood and later adulthood. (The role of family dynamics in the incidence of sexual abuse will be discussed in Chapter 13.)

As a child, Rose began to internalise the fact that she was "bad and dirty", not only because of the sexual abuse but also because of her mother's constant references to the evils of sex, of which of course she was, in her own mind, the (coerced) recipient. The manner in which her father had "initiated" her into sex left her with traumatic memories that were to haunt her until she came to therapy. These became particularly prominent from the time she went to her doctor to request help, and presented themselves in the form of disturbing images, dreams, and sudden flashbacks whenever certain cues or relevant stimuli occurred. Her inability to continue sex therapy with Relate was due to her distress at becoming increasingly unable to disentangle reality from fantasy. In this sense, Rose's sexual abuse experience had established in her symptoms that were compatible with post-traumatic stress disorder, which in addition to the disturbing images, included generalised anxiety, hypervigilance (particularly towards her daughter's safety), avoidance, obsessive compulsive behaviour, and latterly clinical depression. This well recognised syndrome in some survivors of sexual abuse (see Chapter 5) was superimposed on the more enduring personality difficulties that were discussed in the initial formulation.

As a child, the fact that she was unable to comprehend her painful and frightening experience, together with the unavailability of an adult who could comfort, support, and protect her, gave rise to adaptive (albeit, unhelpful) behaviours. The discovery that by scratching and cutting herself on her arms and the inside of her legs, she could make the "noises in her head" stop, became a repeated pattern, usually following her father's advances, and also when her mother would verbally insult her. This behaviour significantly reduced after she left home, but threatened to re-emerge at the time she sought help. This self-destructive behaviour was being replaced by compulsive house cleaning and an obsessive need for order and tidiness. These behaviours exemplified Rose's inability to set appropriate personal boundaries, her attempts at exerting control, and her excessive need towards unattainable perfection as a means of "cleansing herself" and redeeming her perceived flaws as a human being. Indeed, Rose believed she had basic defects that made her socially undesirable and she went to great lengths to avoid situations where she might have to be amongst people.

Rose's feelings of inferiority were not only related to the sexual abuse. She also experienced a lengthy period of bullying at secondary school. Word had got around that the family were fanatical about religion, and gradually her mother's outspokenly critical behaviour deterred Rose's friends from going to visit her. When she found sufficient courage on one occasion to mention the bullying to her mother, the latter added insult to injury by telling her it was her fault for wanting to be friends with these teenage "fallen" girls and she did well to stay away from them. In adult life, Rose found it difficult to enter any room without feeling a sense of shame, defectiveness, and mistrust towards other people. It was only when she decided to do a nursery nursing course, started to make friends, and realised that she was capable in her chosen vocation, that she began to build enough courage to leave home and take a nanny's position abroad. During the therapy sessions, she realised that another reason that prevented her leaving home early was that she was waiting for her sister, who was four years younger than her, to leave home. It had only just struck her how much she feared for her sister's safety, not only in terms of her mother, but also her father.

Therapy plan

Rose's most pressing therapeutic needs, in terms of my formulation, fell into two categories: those that required immediate medical and psychological action, and those that would constitute our work towards the sexual abuse and unhelpful schema resolution. As Rose's old defences began to break down, she experienced very low mood, and although not suicidal (her daughter was too important for her to contemplate such action), she was subjectively and objectively very depressed and I considered that the biological symptoms needed to be treated in order that she would be able to attend adequately to the demands of the therapy. Other immediate interventions included the monitoring of self-harm intent and instruction in alternative methods of stress release; cognitive/behavioural training to deal with negative automatic thoughts and avoidance of pleasurable activities arising from depression; and evaluation of the extent of Rose's compulsive cleaning behaviour and application of CBT techniques.

Once Rose's mood had sufficiently lifted, sexual abuse and schema resolution would begin. Unhelpful patterns relating to subjugation and self-sacrifice, unrelenting standards, emotional deprivation, defectiveness, and social exclusion would also be addressed. Rose's presenting problem of wishing to have a healthy and enjoyable sexual relationship with her husband was not forgotten, but Rose realised that this was no longer the most pressing issue and that it would be addressed when she felt ready.

CHALLENGE: PERSONAL GOALS AND THE "GARDEN GATE"

Rose's engagement in the therapy had become truly established by session twenty. Our collaborative work in an attempt to alleviate her depression, feelings of guilt, and sense of failure, made Rose realise that she had the capability of being in charge of herself in an effective manner. She was now able to trust me and reacted to my direction and confrontation, when needed, in a much reduced defensive manner. In my mind, she was beginning to take the first steps towards her emotional growth. The daunting moment for her arrived, however, when she acknowledged that it was time to deal with the sexual abuse. Although her mood was much improved, the nightmares and flashbacks continued, and she had gained sufficient insight to realise that her overprotective behaviour with her daughter was not healthy. At a review session to discuss Rose's goals for the next stage in therapy, she listed the following:

1. Ease up on her relentless housework.
2. Communicate better with her husband.
3. Improve her self-esteem and learn to mix with people.
4. Improve her maternal skills.
5. Come to terms with the sexual abuse and improve her sexual relationship.

Given Rose's increased level of self-efficacy and the fact that she was now conversant with the problem-solving approach we had been using, I considered that her goals could now be addressed within the next level of therapy, and the principles of the schema-focused work were explained to her. Our discussion of the specific unhelpful patterns that dominated Rose's life gave her a coherent explanation for the reasons she had adopted certain behaviours that were directly relevant to the goals she had outlined. Indeed,

I reassured her that each success she experienced would positively affect other areas in her life. Within this context, there is no clear demarcation between the management of the different goals because they are frequently interconnected.

Rose was particularly able to relate to the fact that her schema of "unrelenting standards" was a self-defeating one in that she never seemed to achieve the excellence she was constantly seeking (goal one). She volunteered that this explained her anxiety about keeping a "perfect" household in an effort to make herself feel better, which of course never happened, and the cycle of unrelenting striving continued. More importantly, in expanding our discussion about this particular schema, she was able to identify not only that her obsessive behaviour had several functions, but also that it had important links with her other schemas of social exclusion and subjugation, and of course her experience of sexual abuse. She realised that in being constantly occupied with housework she could, at least temporarily atone for her feelings of defectiveness. Those very "angry" hands I had noted from the start, reflected her constant need for cleanliness and use of detergents in her quest for the "purity" she felt she lacked and which made her shun the company of others, feeling that she was somehow contaminated. But most of all, Rose was suddenly struck by the fact that by being constantly busy, she was attempting to "block out" very disturbing images and flashbacks, and could also feel "safe" in the knowledge that she was too busy to speak about the abuse. Another realisation was that she had, from an early age, put the well-being of her sister before her own and said it was now clear to her why she had chosen to be a nanny. Being constantly vigilant about the care of those she loved, she could distance herself from paying attention to her own needs, because after all she was worthless and was not entitled to nurturing.

These connections had a powerful impact on Rose, not only in terms of providing her with a coherent way of making her own formulation of her difficulties, but also because she appreciated that her current insight would start the process of "weakening" the very schemas that she felt had provided her with a way of coping with life. There was a moment of acute fear when Rose realised that the goals she had set for herself constituted immense challenges. This moment activated her schema of emotional deprivation and, for the first time since I had met her, she gave off a distinct air of vulnerability and started to cry. She said, "I should be grateful for knowing, at last, that there is an explanation to all this and that I can do something about it, but I am so terrified. If I give up altogether what I've been doing, how will I stay sane? . . . Who will be there to look after me?"

While saying this, Rose had assumed the posture of a small child as she curled her body, placed her head on her lap, and drew her arms over her head. Instinctively, I went to her and put my arms around her. Without saying anything, we stayed in this position, while Rose continued to weep with silent sobs. This was a very crucial moment in the therapy because, at last, Rose could finally start to get in touch with her vulnerability and her needs, and begin the process of realising that trust is possible and it is safe to ask for comfort in a safe environment. At this very moment she had emotionally connected with the needy child inside, and her mother's failure to empathise and protect her came into relief. The way had begun to be paved for the work on her emotional deprivation and the processing of her feelings towards her mother. More importantly, for the remainder of this particular session we looked at ways in which Rose could begin to address her emotional and practical needs at home within a framework of appropriate personal boundaries and limits. For example, when in need of physical comfort, she could start practising asking her husband to hug her without this having to constitute an advance towards sexual behaviour (goal two). Rose was puzzled by this and said, "But don't you think that one thing could lead to another? . . . I mean, men are like this, you give them a little and they want more!" Rose's comment opened up a particularly effective discussion which managed to initiate the start of her personal goal challenges and their achievement. It would be worth paying close attention to the discussion that follows because it exemplifies the subtle connections that link one particular targeted area (by Rose) with another. More importantly, it provides a good example about how the current dynamic (at home and in therapy) can be used as a vehicle towards change.

I picked up her comment by saying: "Rose, what makes you think that by asking Tony to hug you, he will expect to also have sex with you?" She thought about this for a while and then said, "Well, now you ask I'm not sure, as I've never really been the one to go to him for a hug. In fact, Tony is the affectionate one, but I seem to always push him away . . . making excuses that I'm in the middle of something." I responded by saying, "You have no proof then that Tony will want more if you just wanted some affection . . . What made you think he would?" The conversation was clearly causing Rose to think very hard and it was some time before she said, "You know, I've never really given it much thought . . . well, not in so many words, it was just a feeling. . . . You see, there was never any form of physical touching in my family . . . well certainly not from my mother." At that point Rose looked distinctly uncomfortable, as though she had made some important realisation, and started to cry. She continued talking and said, "My father was the only man other than Tony to touch me, and look what he did. . . . My, so called, monster of a father has actually ruined my life. . . . I've only just realised that I had tarnished all men with the same brush. I seem to have forgotten that I actually chose Tony because he's always been so gentle and kind. I know he misses being close to me and always shows me how much he cares in different ways. . . . What am I doing to him . . . to all of us?"

These connections must have had a cathartic effect because Rose continued to cry for a while, but the sense of relief she felt was quite tangible. My reply to Rose consisted of, first, acknowledging that she was right to be confused about how she was behaving towards her family; then, I illustrated my observation using the metaphor of the "garden gate". This metaphor has evolved during the course of my work with survivors and I have used it very frequently because it succeeds in providing a good conceptual understanding of the importance of personal boundaries, which helps to regulate our behaviour towards others and also the behaviour of others towards us. I said: "We all need an invisible gate around us that has a door bearing a sign which says either, 'open' or 'closed'. Note that this is not a huge barrier which does not allow us to see what lies beyond, but one that gives us a good view of the world around us. The sign also allows us to invite in what we want from the outside world, or indeed, to keep it away from us if we so wish. From the time we are small children, our parents or those who care for us have the responsibility of helping us, not only to start erecting our own gate but also observing the signs on other people's gates. This takes great care, love, guidance, and if need be, helpful confrontation; but most of all, it requires that the carer or parent respects and tries to understand our individuality and what our needs are. This also means that the parent or carer must never abuse their position of authority by crossing over to the child's 'gate' or boundary. Unfortunately this is the ideal position, and while a lot of parents or carers try to do their best, others neglect this important duty or do it in a haphazard fashion, and another group actually disrupt the whole 'gate building' process by walking straight into the child's space. This is the case with sexual, physical, and emotional abuse."

Rose listened with great attention to what I was saying, and I had already anticipated her question, which was, "What you've just said explained exactly what happened to me when I was a child, and why it is that now I don't know how to behave, and how wrong it was what my father and mother did to me . . . but it is also scary. . . . I haven't got this 'garden gate'. . . . So what now?!" My response signalled the beginning of real hope in Rose that she could now start to be the master of her own behaviour and, therefore, her life. I said, "Rose, this is why you are here. Together, we will start the process of creating a new 'gate'. Remember I said to you a while ago that, as a therapist, at times I need to act as a parent in a limited way. My responsibility is to help you start creating your own personal boundaries that will help you to know which are the things that are right for you and your family, and which are the things to avoid. We will do this by talking, by carrying out certain exercises, and by creating experiments to see if some of the things we discuss actually work in real life. I know it will not always be easy, but it is the challenges you are prepared to take and the feeling that you have succeeded in controlling your life in helpful ways that will give you the greatest satisfaction and self-confidence. . . . Remember, this time you are not alone."

RELEVANCE OF BOUNDARY SETTING AND SUMMARY OF THERAPEUTIC STRATEGIES

The actual sexual abuse resolution and the management of Rose's sexual relationship with her husband will be accorded individual discussion in a separate section below. Here, I will discuss the relevance of the points raised in the preceding sessions with Rose, with reference to her tackling challenging tasks in order to meet her personal goals.

The explanation given to Rose about personal boundaries, within the "garden gate" metaphor, had the following beneficial effects. First, it began to allay some of the feelings of responsibility she had assumed about the fact that her father had sexually abused her, because she was able to understand his failure in maintaining appropriate parental boundaries (goal five). Secondly, she was also able to start comprehending that she was not to blame for the fact that her mother did not treat her with respect and love, and that it was the latter's responsibility to teach and guide her about life, as well as help her create a solid identity base. Indeed, she expressed huge surprise that she had not appreciated these issues earlier while training as a nursery nurse. As part of her course material there was a section that dealt with appropriate parental attitudes, and one looking at certain behaviours/signs in small children that might be related to the possibility of there being abusive behaviour at home. Her explanation was that she had managed to block her own experience while focusing totally on the well-being of others. She realised that it was only when she saw "in action" the behaviour of families she had worked with that she started the process of comparison with her own family. When discomfort really set in, she had already met her husband and given up her work. Her real distress started after she had her daughter and, of course, when she began the process of seeking help for her sexual difficulties.

This realisation had direct relevance to the work we started to do in relation to her goal of improving her self-esteem (goal three). The "garden gate" metaphor was extended to explain that good self-esteem is directly proportional to the degree that we are able to ensure that we have skills of self-knowledge about who we are and what we need (either emotionally or physically) and that we are able to regulate, through assertiveness as well as intuition, "incoming" and "outgoing" events in our life. Because Rose was not taught these skills, our task was to do just that through a variety of experiential as well as cognitive/behavioural tasks, particularly rehearsal, and mostly identification of personal needs and schema dialogue in relation to subjugation (see Jehu, 1988; Fennell, 1997; Young, 1994).

The work on her self-esteem was linked to our work on tackling her feelings of defectiveness and social exclusion. Using these, Rose was able to identify the origins of these schemas and get in touch with her feelings of defectiveness as a child and her social exclusion at school, due to the bullying and also the lack of nurturing at home. The combination of schema confrontation, gradual establishment of appropriate personal boundaries, and more desirable self-image, allowed Rose to feel more confident about undertaking certain challenges that required meeting new people. One such example was her agreement to start taking "risks" when collecting her daughter from nursery by initiating conversation with other mothers. In other areas of social interaction, the garden gate metaphor proved particularly useful to Rose in negotiating her own as well as other people's responses, always referring to her now more alert understanding about her needs and those of others.

Her level of self-confidence was particularly enhanced by her understanding of personal boundary setting, in that she was able to apply this knowledge in her role as mother, which was another one of her stated aims (goal four). By being vigilant about how she used her love and care of her daughter in helping her start her own process of "garden gate" setting, she was able to realise that her excessive vigilance over her daughter's safety was not helpful in promoting self-confidence, self-reliance, and therefore social skill in later life. For example, Rose would not allow anyone to collect her daughter from nursery—not even her grandmother (Tony's mother)—even though she had no reason not to trust her, and actually got on very well with her. Moreover, she had maintained that she would never allow her daughter to go to her friends' homes once she went to school because, "you never know what might happen" (meaning the possibility of abuse). During the course of the work that we were doing, however, this excessive vigilance was discussed and the process of confronting her mistrust in a realistic manner, as well as education about appropriate boundaries for a child, and the teaching of self-protective techniques, addressed Rose's goal of being a more relaxed and effectively protective mother.

During the course of this work, we were also able to use the contrasts between Rose's new approaches with her daughter and those of her own mother, in addressing her goal of coming to terms with the latter's behaviour. Most of all, Rose began to understand the effects that the lack of warmth, love, and protection had on her as a person and also in her relationship with Tony. During the process of "unsent letter" writing, schema confrontation (emotional deprivation), and role-play she was able to identify her counter-productive behaviours that perpetuated her feelings of "unlovability" and isolation; once she was prepared to take small "risks" with Tony, such as letting him see her vulnerability and allowing him to comfort her by talking to her and hugging her or holding her, a significant breakthrough was realised towards completing the resolution of sexual abuse and its effects.

SEXUAL ABUSE RESOLUTION

The most difficult challenge for Rose was to actually talk about, describe, and then attempt the tasks towards resolving the memory of her abuse and the current images that haunted her. We carried out this work once her depression had substantially subsided and she had started making gains in some important practical areas in her current life (see earlier discussion). For this task we used the techniques of written accounts of the abuse; guided imagery with rescripting; unsent letter writing; and joint therapy with her husband.

Personal accounts

I have already mentioned that Rose's personal account was one of a number she wrote in order to begin the challenging process of cognitive and then emotional processing. At this stage, I am taking it for granted that the reader appreciates that the level of engagement and trust between therapist and survivor has reached a point that inspires the survivor with a degree of confidence and safety. Goodwin (1997), in a paper that discusses CSA sequelae, argues that various professionals' clinical experience suggests that one very important aspect of recovery is related to "telling the story". This is because the survivor needs to be believed concerning all aspects of their story, and in so being, feelings of self-blame, disgust, and of being alone may begin to be addressed and healed. Moreover, in Rose's case, the long-term effects of her very traumatic experience were not dissimilar, in terms of PTSD features, to those experienced by women who have been raped (see Jehu, 1991; Resick and Schnicke, 1993).

Within the context of these complex difficulties, the process of repeated "story" writing had several benefits for Rose. First, it enabled her to start putting into words something she had not spoken about in detail to anyone, and it allowed her a degree of safety from having, in the first instance, to verbalise her ordeal in a face-to-face situation. Secondly, the sheer repetition of the accounts served as an "exposure" exercise that began to reduce the excessive levels of anxiety and fear that Rose had been negatively affected by for several years, as well as significantly reduce the frequency of flashbacks and intrusive images.

Thirdly, her accounts provided us with invaluable information about the specific events, memories, or other cues in her experience of rape by her father, which constituted the material for her very distressing flashbacks and recurring images. This identification was facilitated by the instruction given to Rose that she should underline any section she had written that proved to be particularly difficult for her and which aroused unpleasant emotions. This task allowed us to subject any remaining intrusions to more in-depth cognitive/emotional processing, which had the fourth benefit of highlighting a key event in Rose's experience that later formed the "scenario" for our guided imagery task. The latter was instrumental in the overall and vital completion of the emotional processing or "digesting" work, which reversed her feelings of powerlessness. Finally, our work was directly relevant to the schema-based work we later carried out in relation to her perception of her husband's intentions, her negative feelings about sex, and the couple's sexual relationship.

Guided imagery

The event that Rose found most traumatic and, therefore, most difficult to come to terms with was the one in which she had been "initiated" into her sexual ordeal with her father. The recurring images that haunted Rose presented themselves to her as follows: First, she would have a picture in her mind of the time when she was ill in bed on that fateful Sunday when everyone else had gone to church. Then, she would see her father as a large looming figure towering over her, holding in one hand the cup of hot chocolate he had brought to her, as she was lying on her bed. Mostly, she had succeeded in stopping the images at that particular point, but latterly— particularly since the time we had started to address her compulsive cleaning and self-harm—she found to her great distress that she could no longer halt the rest of the image. The second part of her image consisted of her seeing herself as a tiny figure on the bed being squashed by the enormous weight, which was her father; in her words: "I am lying in bed, feeling like a normal little girl one minute, then this huge figure comes over me and it feels like a big black cloak is swallowing me, the next. . . . I feel terrified, and then I feel as though a sword is being pushed between my legs and cuts me in half. . . . When it's all over my father is lying next to me crying. . . . I'm so confused and scared. . . . I don't know what to do. . . . I just want to die."

Rose's feelings of confusion and fear, physical pain, betrayal, but mostly powerlessness, are acutely expressed in her own words. Moreover, this haunting image clearly illustrates the manner in which a memory is encoded in very basic symbols that represent the host of emotions a child experiences in such traumatic circumstances. Indeed, so powerful was this image for Rose in terms of its representation of the emotional content of her traumatic experience, that in the absence of maturity and intellectual ability to make sense of the events, together with a consistent lack of appropriate adult warmth, protection and guidance, as was the case for Rose during her childhood, it recurred during her adult life as testimony to its enduring qualities, which was to remind her that part of her was still stuck at age nine. More crucially, it was a constant reminder of her lack of power to change the events of the past, which rather than positively spurring her to overcome the ordeal, compounded her feelings of failure and self-disgust.

Rose had already been briefed about the fact that we would carry out a guided imagery task, when we both felt she was ready to do so. The time at which Rose felt ready for the exercise was when she had written four accounts of her ordeal; the repeated exposure to this painful material had helped Rose to make substantial progress. Moreover, the gains she had already made in other areas provided her with the necessary strength and resolve to face up to her demons head on. We carried out imagery tasks with rescripting that were broken down into three stages.

Stage one

With her eyes closed, Rose was guided to talk through the image that had been the most haunting for her (see above). She was also instructed to describe the image in the present tense, while retaining her present adult identity outside the imagery. She said she saw herself in bed with her father approaching her, holding a cup of hot chocolate. Then she saw him coming towards her and was guided to stop the image just before he was about to get into bed with her. Rose was also encouraged to elicit memories in all sensory modalities in order to make the image as real as possible. She said that she could hear no sounds as the house was very still but could just make out the sound of her father's breathing which became deep and heavy as he was approaching her bed. She could feel the warmth of her bedclothes around her and could detect a faint smell of sweet hot chocolate. At one point she opened her eyes saying that she had just realised why she had never been able to drink hot chocolate since that time. She was also able to express intense sadness at the fact that this symbolised her lost childhood and that she was never able to experience the innocent comfort which drinking hot chocolate could bring (survivors are guided to make a sign at any stage during the imagery task if they wish to stop; this can be done by lifting a finger or raising the hand).

In the first stage of the task "little" Rose was guided to imagine an adult person in the room and call upon her/him to help her stop her father from getting into bed with her. She asked if this person could be myself as she could not think of anyone else she trusted and did not feel that enlisting her husband's help would be "authentic" enough. We had previously discussed that the aim of the imagery was for Rose to regain power by stopping her father from abusing her, and she had expressed her concern that she would not be able to do this as she felt too small and vulnerable. The latter spontaneous observation alone had a significant impact on Rose because it succeeded in confirming our previous discussions about the fact that she was not responsible for her father's actions. For some survivors, reaching such a stage is sufficient in absolving their misplaced feelings of guilt and responsibility. It can also help them in deepening their insight and understanding that while they may have been vulnerable in childhood and that it is a parent's full responsibility to observe boundaries, they can nevertheless be empowered in later life. In some instances, however, as was the case with Rose, it is important to "rescript" the image in order to reverse the deeply entrenched perception of powerlessness that perpetuates itself into adulthood. After showing the nine-year-old Rose that another adult can successfully intervene in stopping her father from abusing her (in this case myself), we progressed to the second stage.

Stage two

In the next stage of the imagery tasks, Rose was encouraged to stop the abuse by taking two parts in the task. One was still to be herself as the nine-year-old Rose in bed, and the other was to be her adult self as she currently was. She was to stand by the bed and ask her father to stop from getting into bed with "little" Rose because what he was about to do was wrong. Rose found this task initially very difficult and said that she was not sure whether she could stop her father even as an adult. We discussed this for a while and I suggested that I could stand at the back of the room as a protective and supporting influence while she did so, and when she felt sufficiently confident then I could leave the room. This was a successful tactic and the "adult" Rose was able to stop her father from abusing "little" Rose.

Stage three

In the third stage of the imagery, "adult" Rose was to carry out the task of stopping her father from abusing "little" Rose without additional help. Once again, the adult Rose felt very concerned that her upbringing had been such that she was "not supposed to contradict her parents". This statement represented Rose's final link to her feelings of powerlessness and, once I reminded her of the "garden gate" analogy and the fact that she had the right to expect appropriate boundaries, she was able to carry out the final part of the imagery.

A word of caution and final resolution

Guided imagery exercises may seem straightforward enough, but it must be borne in mind that I have provided the reader only with basic information about the procedure. To have gone over every single detail of the preparation towards this exercise would have constituted a whole separate chapter, and this has not been one of the aims of this book. Although I have provided a reading list in the Appendix, it cannot be stressed enough that anyone undertaking such exercises must have extensive experience and confidence in their work as a therapist, particularly with survivors of sexual abuse. If in training, regular supervision must be sought from someone who is skilled in such procedures.

For the current purpose, the guided imagery discussion was included in order to illustrate that feelings of powerlessness in survivors of sexual abuse must be addressed in a medium of therapy that succeeds most in reversing such feelings. For Rose, in particular, the guided imagery with rescripting had a very positive and even fundamental outcome towards the resolution of the effects of her abuse. It provided her with a new, solid base on which to continue her work of personal boundary building, and more importantly it created the necessary conditions for the work on her presenting problem—that of her sexual relationship with her husband. She had now reached a stage where she was able to perceive herself as an adult woman who had the right not only to stipulate certain needs, but also one who had the ability and confidence to repel those things that she did not want. Although apprehensive about the prospect of sex therapy with her husband, she was sufficiently reassured that this was a two-way negotiation in which she would have her own appropriate control. Indeed, the combination of our guided imagery work and the graduated exposure to sex therapy exercises once her husband became involved in joint sessions, had the required effect of gradually extinguishing the disturbing images with which Rose had been so troubled. The sexual abuse had now been finally relegated to the past and she was able to focus on her present life, which, for once, provided her with a sense of future.

When possible and appropriate, partners must be included in the process of sexual abuse resolution, particularly if the couple's mutual sexual satisfaction is being undermined by the experience of abuse. There are periods during therapy with survivors when their partners feel shut out from this process and can feel helpless about not knowing how best to be supportive (Firth, 1997). Indeed, during the process of boundary setting with a survivor there can be problematic instances within a couple's relationship that could upset the status quo of power dynamics. When this occurs it is important to suggest joint sessions with a partner, which could be very beneficial not only with respect to sexual difficulties but also to the general equilibrium of the couple's relationship.

The resolution of sexual abuse inevitably involves questions related to the survivor's future involvement with their perpetrator and also the family as a whole. This issue is discussed separately in Chapter 13. In Rose's case, she decided that although she had made substantial progress in coming to terms with the failure of her parents to give her an adequate start to life, she had no wish to resume any kind of contact. She decided, however, to make some effort in contacting her brother towards whom she had harboured anger as well as sadness about the fact that he had "abandoned" her and also her sister. This proved to be a positive decision and she was, eventually, able to disclose her abuse to him and her reasons for not responding to some of his earlier attempts to get in touch with her. She was surprised and also very gratified to hear him say: "It's terrible you know, but somehow I'm not surprised. I always felt that our family was odd and that's why I couldn't wait to get out of there. Now I'm so sorry that I was too immature and angry to stay and help out".

As far as her sister was concerned, she had always maintained a close relationship with her even though the latter lived at some geographical distance away. She had always harboured a fear that she too may have been abused by their father and it was only towards the end of her therapy that she found the courage to ask her and also disclose her own abuse. The fact that her sister had not endured this experience had a profound effect on Rose because she was able to strengthen the feelings of her progressive empowerment by realising that at least her efforts towards protecting her sister had succeeded and that all her suffering had not been in vain.

In order to put a closure to the abuse resolution, Rose decided to send one of the "letters" she had written to her father, as part of our therapeutic work. We discussed this at length and weighed up all the pros and cons of sending the letter, and Rose felt that, while she had no wish to confront her mother, she felt that the gains she had so far achieved deserved a fitting closure. She was also able to volunteer that in sending this letter she was not expecting some miraculous repentance from her father, but that she was doing so for her own benefit in that she wanted him to know the destructive effects of his actions and, most importantly, the fact that she had overcome these and was finally enjoying life. While telling me this, she was even able, for the first time in her therapy to make a joke that spoke volumes about the level of freedom and growth she had reached. With a smile that expressed her self-contentment, she said: "The best type of revenge is success!" The final version of the letter she sent to her father went as follows:

Dear father
I'm not sure why I'm calling you this as you don't deserve the title, but nothing can change the fact that you brought me into this world. I should have been precious to you, and I should have had your love and protection, the type that a proper father gives to his daughter. Now I understand fully how you failed to give me a good start in life by showing me how to respect and like myself and guiding me to be a confident and successful human being. Your actions were monstrous and made me feel very afraid and then very dirty and disgusting. You also made me feel confused and I thought I must have done something to deserve this

treatment. You also let me and my sister down by not protecting us from our mother's foul temper and the strange ways she had about talking to us about life and other people. Had I not met Tony, my husband, who knows what would have become of me as I would have never thought to get help if I was just on my own. . . . I would have never felt I was worthy of help. But he and my baby daughter made me realise that I had to do something before I destroyed their lives as well. I have been receiving professional help for some time and now I can finally see a future for myself and my family. I am also beginning to really like myself and realise that, like other people, I too have talents of which I can be proud. Most import-antly, I have been helped to see that I was not responsible for what you did and that it was fully your responsibility when you decided to cross a forbidden boundary. I have hated you for a long time and never thought I would be able to write to you, but now I must put the past behind me, and I have decided that I must let you know what you did and what effect this had on me. I no longer hate you but feel very, very sorry for you and also for my mother. I don't know what happened in your own childhood, but it cannot have been a very happy one, or else why would you have done what you did? I am not writing this letter to punish you, for what good would this do? It is up to me to make the hurt stop and I now know I can do this. I have written to you because I need to leave what happened to me in the past and I also need to tell you that you have not managed to destroy my life. I have no wish to see you or mother again as I know that this will not be good for me. I have a feeling that you prefer this too, or else why is it that neither of you tried to find out where I am? I hope that now I have written to you, you may start to think about what you did and then find some kind of peace in yourself. I do not wish you or mother any harm, and although I will never forget, I am able to leave the past where it belongs and, therefore hold no malice towards you both. Goodbye.

CONCLUDING SESSIONS: INDEPENDENCE AND GROWTH

Rose's therapy was spread over the best part of two years, and this was followed by a few monthly and then quarterly follow-ups. Her move towards independence and growth had of course started the moment she entered therapy, but this became particularly visible when she gained sufficient trust to be able to collaborate in the very challenging tasks that her therapy demanded. With each gain Rose made, she began to flourish from the state of angry, frightened child, to confident and capable adult.

To nurture and guide Rose through these difficult stages was immensely challenging, and, inevitably, as the limited parent, my fondness for Rose grew and I felt almost as though she was my own child. It is this form of genuine empathy that provided Rose with the trust and courage she needed in order to put the monsters of her past to sleep. For my part, I had to be vigilant (as I always am) about the need for an appropriate boundary between my role as therapist and that of limited parent. My involvement with Rose, as with all survivors, kept me alert to the fact that our relationship would be coming to an end and that I must competently pave the way towards independence. During the course of our reviews towards the end of her therapy Rose would frequently comment that she did not know how she would cope without her sessions with me. We spent a great deal of time addressing Rose's anxieties about "separation" and in so doing Rose was able to acknowledge that, actually, she no longer needed me to "show her the way" and that she was confident with the manner in which she was now conducting her life. She realised that her anxiety revolved around the fact that "losing me" would be like losing a safety net, in that there would be no one to guide her when things went wrong.

Her perceived fears initiated us into the very important closing stages when survivors detach from their therapists and realise that they no longer need them because they have sufficient resilience and confidence in their own self-guidance. Indeed, this realisation is the final and most important stage to reach as it brings to fruition the whole course of therapy towards independence and perceived competence. The closing stages in therapy must be handled with great care because each survivor presents with differing levels of anxiety and apprehension about ending contact with their therapist. In Rose's case, we agreed to distance the sessions by several weeks, as an experiment to see what types of anxieties, if any, she would have. Rose was to keep a diary of the latter and I also suggested she could contact me by phone, only if it was absolutely necessary. This was a fruitful exercise as Rose was able to report that, apart from having fleeting twinges of anxiety about not seeing me, she was able to use the coping strategies we had discussed. Keeping a diary and subjecting her anxieties to cognitive challenge, confirmed the fact that she was able to deal with these quite effectively, thus increasing her feelings of self-competence. In addition, the fact that she was now able to share her concerns with Tony as well as be comfortable in asking for warmth and reassurance, made her realise that her practical and emotional needs could be fulfilled by herself and those closest to her, and that I was not indispensable. Possibly the greatest realisation Rose made was that now it was she who was the "garden gate" setter in her role as parent and that it was her responsibility to convey to her daughter an example of competence, strength, and independence. So delighted was Rose with this realisation that she suggested our monthly follow-ups be reduced to quarterly meetings with a view to ending by the close of the third year in therapy.

I had only two communications from Rose following the end of therapy. One was when she sent me a card and a bouquet of flowers to thank me for helping her "find herself" and also a future. The second time I heard from her was about a year after I had last seen her when she telephoned me to say that she was pregnant with her second child, that all was well, and that she had been in part-time education towards a degree. She sounded like a woman who was excited by what life had to offer and who was positively enriched by the opportunities that education brings, both academically and socially. Rose's maturity, freedom from "emotional chains", and positive delight at being alive was acutely audible as I was talking to her on the telephone. I was grateful to Rose for that phone call because it was her way of saying, "Here I am a year later and I have made it. . . . I wanted to tell you this because I respect you and think you should know what you have helped me achieve." It is these small but profoundly touching moments for which I am so grateful; they continuously spur me on to do my work as they succeed in providing the best type of feedback any therapist could ever wish for.

FINAL COMMENTS

I chose to tell Rose's story because of the complexity of her difficulties, and considered that the reader would appreciate the insights gained from following her progress in the therapeutic context. Rose is a survivor whose adult life had been substantially affected by her experience of sexual and emotional abuse; subjectively as well as objectively she was a woman whose adjustment to the day-to-day demands of life was "bad" at the time she presented for therapy. I hope that the highlights of Rose's journey towards psychological health and independence have succeeded in bringing into relief the most pertinent aspects of her difficulties and distress. The latter are best understood within the context of three main theories proposed as an explanation of the long-term sequelae. Finkelhor's (1988) traumagenic model is particularly relevant in terms of issues relating to Rose's power-lessness; stigmatisation; traumatic sexualisation; and, of course, betrayal. Her fear and anxiety, perception of poor self-efficacy, as well as her excessive need for control, were at the forefront of her initial presentation and were successfully addressed over the course of our work, which led to her empowerment as an adult woman. The experiential part of the therapy within a schema-based approach was particularly effective in reversing her feelings of powerlessness, and in healing the traumatic sexualisation. The latter was a key factor in helping build a healthy sexual as well as emotional relationship with her husband, as well as helping to reduce the sense of stigmatisation that had led to social exclusion.

In helping Rose it was also important to take note of the fact that the traumatic sexualisation had not only been instrumental in the acquisition of personal maladaptive schemas, but in addition it had a serious psychological impact which could best be addressed using the post-traumatic stress disorder (PTSD) model (DSM-IV, American Psychiatric Association, 1994). This was evident in some of Rose's distressing symptoms such as hypervigilance, intrusive images, anxiety, and avoidance of stimuli which were associated with the traumatic event, namely a sexual relationship with her husband (Smith and Bentovim, 1994). It has also been documented that when sexual abuse involves multiple episodes of intercourse, as was the case with Rose, there is a greater likelihood of PTSD symptomatology (Briggs and Joyce, 1997).

The fact the Rose's perpetrator was her biological father had particular significance in terms of her feelings of betrayal and general insecurity within a household that was lacking in warmth. These types of family dynamics will be discussed in detail in Chapter 13, but suffice it to say that in Rose's case, the situation typified the type of environment where her father looked to his wife for support and had little power to assert himself within the family. His emotional and sexual needs not being met by Rose's mother, together with his impoverished status in the home, created the right conditions for a type of role reversal situation whereby Rose was fulfilling her mother's "duties" (Pelletier and Handy, 1986). One of the difficulties for Rose resulting from this experience was her fear of intimacy with her husband, which is a well documented long-term effect (DiLillo and Long, 1999). On the other hand, her mother's unavailability and lack of empathic understanding of Rose and her needs, did not provide her with the protection and care she required.

This point introduces the third framework completing Rose's theoretical understanding of her difficulties. The developmental model, as was the case with Victoria, helps to explain the dysfunctional family dynamics within which sexual abuse can occur. Cole and Putman (1992), in particular, looked at the long-term effects of abuse in relation to father–daughter incest and suggested that disruption occurs in the areas of self-integrity, self-regulation, and social acceptability, all of which Rose had difficulties with. The reader is reminded about Rose's problems with impulse control and self-destructive behaviour, her insecurity in relation to other people, and her dissociated behaviour in relation to her husband. The developmental model was particularly relevant in defining Rose's problematic schemas in terms of defectiveness, social exclusion, and unrelenting standards. It also helped us to understand the role of her emotional deprivation resulting from the lack of an appropriate bond with her mother and, in so doing, we were able to address the associated disruption to the development of her personality.

I have offered this summary in order to facilitate the process of understanding Rose's complex presentation. This is by no means a finite assessment and I am conscious of the fact that there may exist alternative formulations. The theories I have proposed, however, are the ones that I have found to be most relevant in my work with Rose, and I was able to incorporate them in my integrated therapeutic (working) model. This enabled me to apply a mixture of practical cognitive/behavioural techniques for the more pressing problems, which helped Rose to start gaining a sense of self-efficacy, as well as more in-depth, schema-focused, experiential approaches for the resolution of enduring difficulties resulting from experience of sexual abuse. For Rose, our imagery sessions with rescripting were necessary steps towards empowerment and integration.

Florence

BACKGROUND TO FIRST SESSION

Florence was thirty-six when she attempted her third overdose. The first one was when she was twenty-two and the second when she was thirty, both involving ingesting low doses of paracetamol in combination with alcohol. On both these occasions she telephoned her best friend soon after taking the "cocktail" and was not detained more than one night at the accident and emergency department. She was offered the opportunity of psychiatric and/or psychological help, but she turned down these offers both times, saying it was a "spur of the moment" thing and that she would be perfectly fine.

Her third overdose was much more serious and premeditated. She had been prescribed sleeping tablets by her general practitioner and one evening, after a particularly violent argument with her current boyfriend, she swallowed a moderate amount of paracetamol, and a few sleeping tablets, together with alcohol, and attempted to go to sleep without calling anyone. It was only when her boyfriend returned in the early hours of the morning and wanted to continue the argument with her that he noticed that she appeared to be unconscious and called an ambulance. On this occasion, she was transferred to the psychiatric department after being treated and monitored on a medical ward for a few days. Despite her protestations she was advised to remain in the psychiatric ward for at least two weeks until an assessment of her mental state and appropriate medication were considered. During the course of her stay she was able to talk to her allocated nurse about the difficulties which had led her to want to end her life. She told her that she had been seeing a man for three years and that for the past year he had moved in with her. At first things were fine but he had always been a heavy drinker and in the past six months they had started to have violent arguments and he had, on occasion, hit her across the face. She said that the night she decided to take her own life, he had gone too far, kicking her and using his fists to punch her. She told the nurse that it was like reliving the nightmare of seeing her mother being treated this way by a "monstrous bastard" when she herself was a teenager.

Reluctantly, Florence accepted a diagnosis of depression and agreed to be put on medication but was less agreeable to a suggestion that she would benefit from individual psychological treatment. The staff on the ward were concerned about discharging her given the potential for future violence at home and suggested that she might either want to consider staying else-where or going to a women's refuge until things calmed down. Florence was adamant that she "could handle" her boyfriend, and blamed herself for "pushing him too far" after having a few drinks herself. She said she loved him and wanted to give things another go; after all, had he not been remorseful and come to the ward to ask her forgiveness? When the staff appeared sceptical, she appeased them by promising to curb her drinking and accepting their referral for psychological help.

FIRST SESSION

Florence came to see me on the last day of her discharge from the psy-chiatric ward. She had a very striking presentation. Her looks, the way she was dressed, and also the manner in which she spoke were very much at odds with the information about her in the referral letter. I had expected to see someone who was low in spirits, apprehensive about seeing me, and generally not very happy with life. Florence, on the contrary, was very well and fashionably groomed, and had clearly given a great deal of attention to her hair and make-up. If anything, I thought her make-up was rather heavy for this early time of the day, although it was immaculate and very flattering. She had a beaming smile when she entered the room, and when she sat down and started to speak it was difficult to equate this lively, apparently happy woman, with the one that was described in my notes. Before I even had the chance to ask her anything, she said that she was very pleased to see me as now the staff on the psychiatric ward would "leave her alone", and she hoped that I would write back and say that all was well and that she could cope without needing further appointments. I was, of course, taken aback by her direct and frank approach and felt there was pressure on me to comply to her request. My immediate thought was that Florence was anxious to put across a good impression, but more pertinently at this very early stage, I surmised that Florence was not only very anxious about entering into any deep conversation with me, but also that one of her difficulties was her inability to accept appropriate limits, let alone guidance from anyone. When she finished what she had to say I just looked at her for a while and then very quietly said: "Florence, you seem to want to tell me that there is no reason for you to be here, but the staff on the ward have been clearly concerned about you, so now it is my turn to find out why this is so. It is not easy seeing a psychologist for the first time, and you may be right that there is no reason for you to come back, but I need to ask you a few questions first . . . is this alright with you?"

Florence's initial elation appeared to be suddenly deflated and she sat back on her chair in a resigned manner; she sighed and then said, "I know you're right. . . . I'm sorry. . . . I don't want to interfere with your job, so ask away." There was clearly a defensive tone in her voice and this confirmed to me that the rest of this session would not be easy and that it was crucial to start laying foundations for further contact. My instinct was to respond by saying, "I can't help feeling that you are not at all happy about being here, so this may be a good place to start. Do you want to tell me how it feels?" Florence clearly did not expect this response because at first she looked puzzled then relaxed and seemed to be at ease. She said, "Well, you see, I've always had to look after myself—not to mention other people—and now, suddenly, just because I wanted to end my life, help is coming out of the woodwork. I just can't see how you or anyone else can help me. After all, it's me who's got myself in this mess, so I'm the one who must make sure I get out of it!"

There was an acute sense of anger and resentment in Florence's voice and I responded by saying, "Florence, it seems that you are angry about the help that is being offered to you . . . almost as though it is all too late . . . as though you were once badly let down, is this right?" It was revealing how quickly Florence's mood could switch; one minute she was cheerful and lively; the next she was angry and defensive; and then the next she looked vulnerable and sad. These observations were so telling of the huge efforts she was making to retain a grip on herself, and probably her life. She was also clearly making great efforts not to betray her emotions as she managed a smile and said, "You are absolutely right. It is all too late. I don't really want to die, but sometimes I just get tired from fighting, and when Steve started to hit me, this was the last straw. If someone had helped us when I was small, I would not be in this mess now". She quickly followed this by giving a sarcastic laugh and saying in a jolly tone, "But what the hell Tina, I managed to get here so far, so I should manage at least a few more years, don't you think?" I did not respond to her sarcasm and in a calm but serious tone I said, "I don't yet know what things made you so unhappy in the past, but when someone wants to take their life, then I have a respon- sibility to find out what drove them to such extreme measures. . . . You said it was because Steve hit you, but I can't help feeling there is more to it. Is this right?"

Florence did not reply immediately and appeared to be carefully assess- ing what she was going to say. Eventually she said, "I find it difficult to put things into words . . . you see it is usually a strong feeling of despair that nothing will ever change that makes me do crazy things. I mean, now I think it was mad to try and take my own life, but at the time I felt desperate." I responded by saying, "Florence, can you tell me about other times when you felt such despair?" Florence clearly did not feel comfortable with my question and very quickly said, "I know what you're trying to do. You want me to tell you about the things I've done in the past so that you can tell them 'up there' that I'm crazy and that I need locking up!" I was not expecting Florence to become "personal" so early on in our meeting, and I felt that she was giving me conflicting messages; on the one hand she was volunteering that all had not been well in the past, while on the other she was alerting me to her mistrust of my intentions. I welcomed the opportunity to address our therapeutic relationship and said, "Florence, you are hinting that there are times when you feel very unhappy and desperate, enough to want to take your own life, yet you don't trust me to do the best I can to help you, why is this?"

For the first time in this session, Florence did not attempt to cover up her distress and said, "Why should I trust anyone? I know you probably mean well, but what possible interest could you have in me as a person or what will happen to me in the future? I've met people who got mixed up with psychiatric hospitals and were never the same when they came out". I responded by saying, "Florence, for what it's worth, I may be a professional but I also do care about what happens to you. . . . I also understand that it must feel very lonely not to be able to trust anyone; has it always been this way?" Florence must have got accustomed to my gentle but persistent pressure because she said, "OK, OK. . . . Yes, life has been damned miserable from the moment my father died when I was only nine. From then on I seem to have shouldered the world's problems. My poor mother just fell apart and our once happy family became the family from hell. Who came to help us then? You would have thought that someone at school, or a neighbour, or anyone, would have raised the alarm, but everyone carries on as normal. After I left home, I felt guilty for leaving my mother, but I couldn't stand the memories."

There was so much that Florence was trying to tell me but was clearly finding it difficult. A picture was beginning to emerge of her life and her difficulties, but I felt that we needed to address her suicidal behaviour and ensure that we could come to some contractual agreement that would (a) provide her with coping strategies preventing further attempts at self-harm and (b) instil in her sufficient trust and motivation to return. My response to Florence's last comment was the following: "Thank you for telling me about some of the painful things you've experienced. I hope that we can continue together to look at them and understand how they have affected your life. I don't want to lose sight, however, about the fact that when you are very upset, you think that ending your life is the answer. Can you try and tell me what is the worst thing that drives you to these thoughts?" Clearly, the flow in our communication had begun to ease and Florence said, "I suppose it is when I feel so terribly alone and when everything I try to do doesn't work. . . . Take Steve for example. . . . I've done so much for this man. When I met him, he was out of work, had got himself into trouble with the police, and had no one to care for him. Now he lives in my flat, he has a job, and me to love him, and what does he do? He still drinks too much and now has started to hit me. I just can't cope when he's in one of his moods!" I wanted the momentum of this disclosure to continue and said, "Is it when you feel you've failed at making someone love you that you get so desperate Florence?" She did not hesitate in her reply: "You've got it in one. The last two times I was stupid enough to want to die was when two other cheats decided they were finished with me and moved on. . . . Why do I keep doing this to myself?"

Florence's last comment signalled the beginning of our therapeutic working relationship, albeit within a treacherous and uneven course. At this initial stage, her self-questioning provided the necessary "unlocking" of the barrier hitherto preventing us from addressing her suicidal intent. We were able to discuss in a pragmatic manner the importance of not resorting to such actions and the rationale I used for this was the following: "Florence, I understand now why you feel so lonely and desperate at times and why at such times dying seems a reasonable way to stop the pain. But think of it this way: you say that you have never had anyone you could trust to help you, but now you have the opportunity of such help and although it is still early days and you don't know me that well, would it not be a pity to waste the chance of trying to see if another, less drastic way, could help you not to feel such pain? What I'm saying is, is it surely not worth a try? After all, what have you got to lose?" Florence reflected on my proposal and said: "Well, I suppose when you put it this way it makes sense, but I can't promise anything. You see, these black moods happen all of a sudden and I feel taken over by a strong sense of loss and despair."

Having established however tenuous a link for Florence's next attendance, I used her last comments to involve her in looking at some ways that could be used to reduce the likelihood of being faced with intense and uncontrollable emotions. When I asked her what could she do to prevent such a state, she volunteered that reducing her alcohol consumption would be a good start as she knew that under its influence her emotions were more likely to get out of control. I used her comments as an opportunity to raise the risks of being with Steve, who was a heavy drinker, but at that stage she was not ready to contemplate asking him to move out, but said she knew the women's refuge number if things got "very bad". As a response, I offered to see her together with Steve, but she asserted that there would be no likelihood whatsoever that he would attend because he thought that, "only 'nutters' go to psychologists". In order to put in place a further "safety net", I "contracted" with Florence that she was to ring me if she felt any impulse to self-harm. With these arrangements in place, she agreed to come and see me the following week.

INITIAL FORMULATION

Although I felt as though I had gone some distance in breaking through a few of Florence's barriers, I was in no way confident that she would attend her next session. My experience with survivors of similar presentations left me with no doubt that, were she to return, she would be very difficult to engage in a consistent manner. The initial and most obvious impression I gained was that she exhibited traits compatible with a diagnosis of borderline personality disorder. Her consistent involvement with unstable and rejecting men, which aroused a high intensity of emotion; her affective instability, shifting between irritability, anger, and depression; her impulsive behaviour in terms of alcohol and suicidal behaviour; and her frantic efforts to avoid being abandoned, were all very pertinent in terms of this initial formulation.

More crucially, I detected that beneath Florence's protestations of independence and being able to take care of herself, she was a woman whose main *raison d'être* was to seek connection with another human being, but found herself being thwarted in her efforts by her inappropriate choice of men. Within this context, a very relevant schema to be addressed would be that of "abandonment". Although she did not reveal very much about the nature of her relationship with her father, I was able to detect that he had been very important to her and that his death had had a marked effect on her life. Indeed, the manner in which she described her loss was in terms of a clear distinction between pre-father's death and post-father's death; the first being synonymous with happiness and the second with misery and despair. Consequently, the loss of Florence's father constituted for her a critical event that had not been effectively "processed", and which was continuing to perpetuate unhelpful personal schemas in her attempts to regulate her life.

In Florence's perception, her repeated "failure" to keep a man would ensure that her feelings of loss, abandonment, and inability to reverse the inevitable would become reinforced and act as reminders that she had to "try harder". Given this initial insight, I became acutely aware that Florence's seemingly detached and distant approach towards me could, at a later date, give way to dependence, manipulation, and testing of my reserves to remain as trustworthy as I had claimed to be. This observation helped me to confirm my initial intuition that Florence had difficulty with imposing appropriate limits or boundaries, both for herself and also in her dealings with other people. Not only was she capable of self-destructive behaviour, in terms of her drinking, choice of violent men, and suicidal behaviour, but she could also be the "rebel", who did not have to listen to or respect anyone, and was later to describe herself as a "free spirit". These contrasting shifts, I reflected, could present significant difficulties and I had already prepared myself concerning the importance of remaining vigilant to the task of setting appropriate boundaries and limits, and regulating the "balance of power" between Florence and me. This did not detract from the equally vital task of validating her pain, her fear of abandonment, her fear of connection with anyone, and the clearly painful circumstances of her childhood.

Although Florence volunteered that her mother "fell apart" following the loss of her father, I felt that this alone did not sufficiently explain the emotional intensity with which she referred to the "family from hell" following her father's death. Nor was I totally convinced that her general presentation could be solely accounted for by the loss of her father. I developed a strong suspicion that Florence must have endured some kind of other trauma, and although sexual abuse crossed my mind, I was equally alert to the possibility of neglect and/or domestic violence. Moreover, Florence's frequent angry allusions to the fact that there had been no outside help and her insistence that she had had to rely on her own resources, were strong indicators of the lack of guidance and protection from a stable figure in her life. Significantly, her reference to the fact that she was also responsible to the rest of the family (I knew she was the eldest of three) gave further credence to my initial speculation that she had somehow been placed in a position of responsibility that was beyond her years. This strong possibility highlighted Florence's schema of subjugation, which further explained her need to "rehabilitate" the men in her life at the cost of having her own needs met.

In completing this initial formulation, I also surmised that the schema of mistrust (due to perceived possibility of abuse) would be one that we would need to address. The strength of opposition Florence displayed towards self-revelation, let alone involvement with any professional, was a good indication of her fear and mistrust. It was also an indication that, starting from the moment of her father's death, she gradually lost faith that any adult would be capable of understanding her and helping her. My final cautionary note (to myself), therefore, was to reinforce my previous speculation that the moment Florence started to (hopefully) "open up" would be the moment when the true extent of her unhappiness and despair would unfold, and when her potential for destructive and manipulative behaviour would be at its most active. Under such conditions, creating the balance between appropriate empathy and validation, as well as constructive confrontation, would be of utmost importance.

BACKGROUND TO SECOND SESSION

It came as no surprise when Florence did not attend for her second appointment. I received no message to that effect, nor had she availed herself of my suggestion that she could contact me if she needed to. She had also defaulted on her psychiatric outpatient follow-up appointment. Following my usual procedure, I wrote asking her to get in touch in order to make another appointment, if she so wished. I was tempted to offer her automatically another appointment, but given my formulation regarding "impaired limits" I decided that it was important for Florence to take a certain amount of initiative towards her therapy. Some considerable time passed and I received no reply, and then one day she telephoned me and I could detect that she was inebriated. Her speech was slightly slurred and her voice had a shrill quality in an attempt to put across a jolly tone. She said she was terribly sorry for missing her appointment, explaining, "Hey, you must know what it's like, life gets busy and you forget." When I made no response, she said that she did want to see me again because, "I would be pleased to know" that she had finally kicked Steve out and that she had not fallen to pieces—and then added, "yet".

This type of telephone contact is very difficult because it epitomises all the issues I discussed above. Being presented with such a delicate situation requires one to think "on one's feet" so to speak. Florence had not only defaulted on her appointment without explanation, but she had also disregarded our contractual arrangement about the purpose of telephone calls. She was now presenting me with conflicting messages, saying on the one hand that she had done something positive and was coping, while on the other she was loudly hinting that all may not be well in the future for her. Moreover, she chose to ring me at a time when she had ingested what "sounded" to be substantial amounts of alcohol, which not only transgressed the rule we had contracted, but was also letting me know that in fact she was not coping that well at all. I was immediately made aware that this was my first test and that her future attendance hung in the balance. It was as though she was saying: "Well, you did say you cared, so now I'm showing you what I can be like; what are you going to do about it?"

I was of course aware about her potential towards suicidal behaviour, but at the same time it was important that I did not reinforce this type of behaviour in the future by conveying anxiety or my own potential for being manipulated. In a calm tone of voice, I said to Florence, "I am pleased that you want to come and see me again, and it sounds as though some important things have happened. It would be best that we discuss these at our next meeting". Given her state of inebriation, I surmised that she could quite conceivably forget or misplace the appointment, and before I could say that I would be posting it to her, she said, "So don't you feel proud of me then? . . . I thought you and the others upstairs would be glad that I am shot of the bully. . . . Have you nothing else to say?"

This outburst signalled a dangerous point in this discussion as I felt the future of our therapeutic relationship was hanging on a thread, and yet, if she was to return she would need to have confidence in me as someone who could cope in a crisis and not "lose it", as her mother had done, in her perception. I said, "Florence, I am of course relieved that you are no longer in an abusive situation, but I also know you have been drinking and you yourself know how this can affect you. You can come to see me tomorrow when you have sobered up, but right now I don't think it is a good time to speak." There was silence, and then a more feeble voice answered, "You are right . . . of course you're right. I just wanted someone to know. I'll be there tomorrow."

This is a critical time for a therapist, knowing what a patient is capable of in between sessions, but I have learned that there are always risks to be taken given certain circumstances. Weighing up the current dangers, I considered that the future benefits in terms of Florence's recovery through her ability to trust me to be strong and disciplined were the deciding factors in my response to her first "test" of me.

ENGAGEMENT AND DISCLOSURE

Florence arrived for her session the following day looking very different to the first time I had met her. She had taken little trouble with her appearance and looked as though she had had little or no sleep. She sat down looking somewhat dejected, with no evidence of her previous flamboyant presentation, and waited for me to speak. I said, "Florence I am very pleased you are here. Can you tell me what happened yesterday?" In a rather passive tone of voice she said that Steve had gone "too far" and that he had threatened to kill her if she as much as looked at another man again. They had been out to a party the previous night and Florence became involved in a conversation with a male friend and Steve had accused her of being unfaithful and of making him look like a fool. The following day the argument continued and, after going out and getting drunk, Steve tried to attack her with a kitchen knife, whereupon one of their neighbours, who must have heard Florence's screams, came banging at the door. Steve ran out and she was advised by this neighbour to call the police, but Florence refused. After she finished telling me this she put her head on her lap while crying, and muttering, "What am I going to do? . . . everything is crumbling around me again", and she started rocking her body. I moved closer to Florence and put my arm around her, feeling that the process of her engagement in therapy had started. After a while she composed herself and said, "You know, I always hate people seeing me being feeble and weak, but I now see that unless I start accepting help I will destroy myself and anyone who comes near me. . . . Will you help me?" At this point she started crying again and was sobbing.

Florence's offering of a "truce" in our communication confirmed to me once more that survivors with "impaired boundaries" become more amenable to engagement when they reach a stage of acute subjective distress. I felt as though Florence was now allowing me to probe into her life and, not wishing to waste this opportunity I said, "Florence, please tell me about all those terrible things that happened to you when you were little". She showed no resistance to my very direct question and without hesitating she said, "A bastard posing as my stepfather abused me". Her face creased into a painful grimace and without stopping she continued, "What's more, I had to let him do all those disgusting things to me because he threatened to start on my little sister". At that point she began crying again and said it was a relief to be able to finally "tell" someone because she had kept it under lock and key all these years. She said she had hinted at it to a friend at school but that this friend was going through something similar herself at home and they had made a pact to "kill the bastards" one day. She said, "how could I stoop so low . . . if it isn't enough that I've destroyed my life, and my mother's life. . . . What now?" This was to be a very constructive session and Florence was able to tell me about her grief at losing her father and her attempts to "keep the family going", first after her father died and while her mother was too distraught to cope, and then when she married her stepfather and the domestic violence started. I said to her, "Florence, you seem to have shouldered so much responsibility when you were still so young . . . you must have loved your family so very much". She said, "I was the happiest little girl you could find, until my father died when I was nine, and then I wanted this to continue and keep his memory alive . . . but I failed."

I asked Florence why she felt she had failed, and she said that if she hadn't been frightened by her stepfather's threats that the family would fall apart if she "told", and had found the courage to tell her mother after his first assault on her, then her mother would have thrown him out and they would have continued to be happy and at peace. She then said, "You see, I could have stood his lecherous hands touching me and all the disgusting things he made me do, if everything else was going well and my mother was happy, but none of if did any good. . . . Horrible as it may seem to you, the sexual abuse was not the worst part of it . . . the worst thing was watching my mother being beaten black and blue and my brother and sister looking terrified every time the bully walked into the room."

The accounts that Florence gave, and her feelings of failure and disappointment, were very characteristic of survivors who have a strong subjugation schema and who assume that it is their duty to fulfil other people's needs at the cost of their own. I therefore considered that it was very important to validate Florence's pain as a result of her experiences, as well as address the issue of her personal needs both in the present and future. Capitalising on the current positive wave of Florence's engagement with me, I suggested that before our next meeting she write an account of her "personal story" during the time of her childhood. I suggested that she may wish to start with the more general aspects of her experience and progress to the more difficult ones gradually, if she felt this helped.

EXTENDED FORMULATION AND THERAPY PLAN

Florence's engagement was constant over the next five sessions and we focused our attention on her "personal account" and the manner in which her experiences had affected her life. This information not only confirmed my speculations in the initial formulation, but it also provided me with further insights about which issues would play a crucial part for the next and very challenging stage in Florence's therapy.

I was concerned that possibly the biggest stumbling block to the therapy would be Florence's unresolved grief about the loss of her father, and that it would be crucial to help her attain a state of resolution regarding this loss. The latter appeared to constitute a significant trauma and one that subjectively acted as the underpinning factor to all the troubles that followed. The extent of anger and guilt that Florence had internalised from an early age was such that, in an attempt to obliterate their potent grip they acted as a raging beacon illuminating the route towards self-destruction. What maintained this defeating cycle was Florence's inability to access her innermost feelings, which appeared to have been buried along with her father. All that she could see was that she had been unable, as the oldest child, to carry over her father's responsibilities and safeguard the well-being of the family; in her perception, her greatest unforgivable failure, however, was the fact that she had disgraced her father's memory by being involved in the unspeakable acts of abuse, but mostly by allowing herself to become the type of person that her father would have been very hurt to see. These perceptions had such a hold on her that the pain they generated was at times too much to bear, and in the absence of any other way of obliterating them, she would seek the comfort of alcohol and, in the past, also casual sex. This behaviour acted as a maintaining factor to all of the things she wished to forget and succeeded only in lowering her impoverished self-esteem further. At such times she would be vulnerable and passive, and her need to succeed in reforming someone who could love her in return would be at its most active.

The honeymoon period of her involvement with men who had violent, controlling, and alcoholic tendencies initially succeeded in providing Florence with a sense of purpose and achievement. However, the moment these men relapsed into alcoholism, violence, and control, the inevitable repetition of her nightmares would once more take hold and her despair would be at its greatest. Having lacked the guidance from a stable and secure relationship that would have instilled in her enduring means of integrity and self-control, Florence would, herself, revert to her own rebellious and self-destructive behaviour. The latter would have time-limited gratification, and during it she would be unreachable in terms of any outside guiding influence such as from friends or professionals. Indeed, she had difficulty maintaining close relationships with friends, and would vacillate between establishing immediate and intense contact with her new friendships, and discarding them without a thought the minute she was challenged on any personal matter. This description confirmed my thoughts in the initial formulation, and once more alerted me to the fact that our therapeutic relationship would be far from harmonious, especially when the necessary confrontation began.

Florence's relationship with her mother had particular significance in the development of her difficulties. Indeed, she was unable to create a balance between the intensity of her anger about her mother's apparent lack of strength and ability to regulate the family home and protect her children, and her equally intense love and concern for her. So great was Florence's regard for her mother, that she had rationalised her disappointment and anger about the latter's failure to intervene in the abuse and better still, obliterate the man who caused it, by assuming personal responsibility for all the ills that befell the family. Florence's assertion that the extent of her emotional pain as a result of having a fractured family was infinitely greater than that caused by the sexual abuse had some validity; but, nevertheless, it exemplified further her inability to access her true emotions and perpetuated the avoidance of anxiety that such a revelation might bring in terms of the neglect and violation she had endured.

With a more rounded formulation, I was able to start structuring a therapeutic "path" for Florence, which would of course require her collaboration and commitment. In the sessions that followed her disclosures I responded to Florence's need for validation and support; I considered, also, that it was important to start alleviating some of her guilt by explaining that, while she felt bad about some of the things she had done, she had reasons for doing them and that she adopted them in her attempt to cope and help the family. I took this opportunity to explain the function of unhelpful schemas and how these develop, as well as the emotions and behaviours that they promote. Florence was particularly able to relate to my proposition that it was her feeling of abandonment following her father's death that explained a great deal of her despair when her relationships failed and her guilt that she could not "make any man stay". She was also relieved by my explanation that children have a propensity towards assuming responsibility for their parents when things go wrong, and that her attempts to make "everything better" were understandable. The latter, I explained, created another unhelpful pattern—of subjugation—and that as long as she perpetuated it her feelings of anger and frustration would continue because her own needs for nurturing would never be met. I also addressed with her the intensity of her feelings towards her mother and the fact that she had felt let down by her, especially in terms of the sexual abuse and domestic violence. Once more, I offered the metaphor of "garden gate" or appropriate limits, and acknowledged with Florence that, in the absence of guidance, being a rebel and venting her anger in ways that were not helpful was understandable. Indeed, I stressed to her that working on establishing appropriate boundaries for herself, as well as observing other people's, would be an important first step in her therapy.

During those initial sessions, Florence was clearly relieved to have at last found some explanations about the course that her life had taken, and appreciated my suggestion that finding more helpful solutions rested on her collaboration with me. Indeed, before I even addressed the fact that she would have to seek professional help for her drinking, she volunteered that she would take whatever necessary steps were needed to control her habit.

CHALLENGES AND PERSONAL GOALS: STAGE ONE

Following on from our discussions, Florence had a positive response to my suggestion that it would help if she broke down her therapeutic goals in manageable chunks and, having considered these, she expressed the following:

Short-term
1. Accept help with her drinking.
2. Not allow Steve back in her life.
3. Start looking for another job.
4. Take better care of herself and understand her needs.
5. Write to her mother.

Mid-term
1. Resolve her grief about losing her father.
2. Come to terms with the sexual abuse.
3. Improve her relationship with her mother and siblings.
4. Stop feeling like a failure and improve her self-esteem.

Long-term
1. Learn to develop healthier relationships—with men and friends in general.
2. Go to college.

I had already been alerted to Florence's impatience and her urgency for "quick results", and it was important to explain that success is built in gradual building blocks. Indeed, having considered and written down her goals, she herself volunteered that "staggering" her goals in this fashion made more sense as she would not be able to tackle everything at once. Moreover, we had previously agreed that without first managing her drinking and Steve's potential return, success in the other areas could be severely affected. Florence had admitted that dealing with these two issues presented a great challenge to her, but at that early stage in her "positive" engagement she appeared to be wholeheartedly committed to the task. So much so, that she accepted my referral to the relevant service offering appropriate guidance and advice regarding her drinking. We made a contractual agreement that if she were to resume her drinking her sessions would be suspended until she had abstained for at least two weeks.

With respect to Steve, he had, predictably, attempted to contact her and was full of remorse and promises that he would never again behave the way he had. After her initial resolve, Florence was tempted to take him back and our sessions focusing on all the reasons why this would not be a good idea provided us with a rich and very pertinent background against which to start addressing the schemas of abandonment and subjugation. More importantly, this work allowed us to examine Florence's strong identification with her mother and the incongruity of her conflicted feelings that on the one hand condemned her mother for becoming involved with a violent drunk and on the other allowed herself to contemplate similar relationships. Using the here and now of Florence's circumstances proved to be very fruitful in opening up the journey towards empowerment and improved self-esteem. Indeed, by examining her own motives and subjugation, she was able to begin understanding the complexity of her mother's situation and the difficulty of "doing the right thing" when emotions dictate otherwise. Florence used this insight to fulfil another of her short-term goals, which was to write to her mother. She had broken contact with her more than a year ago and did not respond to any of her mother's letters and telephone calls. It was her own way of punishing her for the past, but this only succeeded in deepening her feelings of guilt towards her as well as her longing for her. Prior to sending her letter, Florence was guided to write a few "unsent" letters in order, in the first instance, to vent her gut feelings. This was for the purpose of catharsis, and most of them, she agreed, would not be suitable to send. The letter she eventually sent read as follows:

Dear Mum
I feel so bad about all the things I've done to you, and miss you so terribly. For years I have blamed you for all the bad things that happened to us from the minute my Dad died. I loved him and you so much and will never forget how happy we used to be until that terrible day when he left us. I wanted you to be strong and help us to carry on as we did before . . . you know, playing games on Sundays, and going for long walks along the river when the weather was good. Dad could be so funny . . . do you remember the funny jokes he used to tell? After he died there was no more laughter in the house and you seemed to fall apart. . . . I didn't know what to do or say to make things better. I thought that if I was good and helped you, then you would start to feel your old self and we would all be happy again. When you met Andy, I hated the idea of another man taking Dad's

place but eventually felt that if this made you happy then it would be worth trying to get used to him. If only you knew what he made me do. For years I was ashamed of letting him use me like a sex toy and felt so guilty about what my Dad would think of me, if only he could see! I know that I once blurted out that Andy tried to rape me, but I knew that you were still weak from all the bad treatment he gave you and I couldn't put more on your plate to worry about. But rest assured that at least I stopped him from doing the worst to me. I was so angry about everything. . . . I think I've been angry all my life and I've only just realised how it has been destroying me. I was angry at Dad for dying and leaving us, I was angry at you for not coping, I was angry at Andy for abusing us, but most of all I think I've been angry with myself.

Mum, I want you to know that I love you and want you to be proud of me. I am sorry for all the bad things I've done to you and for taking all my anger out on you. Now I'm finally getting help, I am beginning to understand how difficult things must have been for you and I don't blame you anymore. I've really missed you and if you can find it in your heart to forgive me, I would like us to start being friends, at least.
All my love, Florence.

Sending this letter represented for Florence an important milestone. Committing herself to paper, as she had done with her personal account, helped her to start accessing the emotions that had so far been deeply buried. Indeed, after sending it she remarked, "It's amazing how a simple thing like writing a letter can clear things up in your head. I can now see what I've been doing and I'm beginning to feel hope that my Mum and I can have a good relationship". Her efforts were rewarded as her mother responded quite promptly and expressed her relief and joy that Florence had forgiven her and that of course she wanted them to be friends, more than anything. After all, was she not her daughter, and had she not always loved all of them, even though she had been too depressed and lost to show it properly. Most importantly, she also told Florence that she was proud of her and that she knew how much she did for all the family and was very, very sorry for what she had to endure with Andy. For what it was worth, she told her she had no idea it was happening, probably because she was too far gone herself in pain and fear to actually notice, and apologised for this.

Having achieved her two initial goals, Florence's self-efficacy began to grow and inevitably her self-esteem also improved, and she felt that she could have a purpose in life. Although very bright, her education had been severely hampered by the domestic events and by her involvement with a group of unruly peers. When I first met her she had been working as a sales assistant but hated the job because she found it too tedious. With her improved self-confidence she registered with several employment agencies and was eventually offered a position as floor manager in a department store, and was overjoyed at being given the opportunity of more responsibility. At this stage of Florence's challenging work, things appeared to be going smoothly and we experienced no "ruptures" in our therapeutic relationship. Indeed, taking stock of these initial successes, Florence collaborated well in cognitive/behavioural tasks aimed towards better self-care through the use of assertiveness techniques, boundary setting, and appreciation of personal needs. As we approached the second stage of our work, which was several months into our therapeutic relationship, Florence's personal circumstances changed and we experienced some ruptures that threatened the flow of our alliance.

CHALLENGES AND PERSONAL GOALS: STAGE TWO

We were to begin working on Florence's unresolved grief about the loss of her father, which was an issue that perpetually cropped up in our sessions but which Florence wished to "contain" until she had achieved her initial goals. She had succeeded in remaining sober for almost a year and had become involved in a relationship with another junior manager in her store. At first all was well, and then one day Florence attended her session in a great state of elation and she even suggested that maybe she did not need to see me anymore. While not wishing to deflate her joy, I was naturally concerned that she was allowing this very recent state of affairs to detract her from the goals she had set for herself, and that she was, once more, avoiding having to face up to some very challenging and pertinent issues. I expressed this to her by saying, "Florence, I am so happy for you, the way you talk about Chris makes him sound like a really nice man. . . . I am not so clear though why you feel you no longer need your therapy?" Florence seemed to sulk a little and then said, "Well, I can't remember when I've been so happy and you must admit, love can conquer all—well, doesn't it? I mean, now I've found someone nice, then everything else may fall into place and I will be able to let my Dad's soul rest in peace." Florence's reply was so in keeping with my earlier formulation regarding her feelings of abandonment and need to find "love" in order to deal with the discomfort it aroused, that I was naturally very conscious about the potential for further disappointment. I said, "Florence, you are right, love is a great thing and it can indeed be very healing—we all need it—I just want you not to lose sight of the fact that the loss of your father still causes you pain and that you must not decide to stop your therapy so soon after meeting Chris."

Florence's sudden shift in mood reminded me of the first time I met her and she reverted to her angry and sarcastic mode by saying, "Well, it's all very well you saying this, and don't get me wrong, I'm grateful for all your help and guidance, but it's not you who has to lie in bed at night feeling lonely and unloved. I just can't stand it anymore. And anyway, it's up to me whether I want to continue or not. . . . it's my life, I should know what's best!" Being acutely aware that this could signal not only a premature, but also very negative end to our therapeutic relationship, I asked Florence to allow me a couple of minutes to think through what she had just said. There was so much that she was trying to convey to me; on the one hand, she was telling me she had achieved a number of things and was now ready to move on, and that she could take care of herself; on the other hand, she was letting me know that she needed love and comforting and was perceiving me as not appreciating this basic need; she was also seeing me as the bearer of bad news and was trying to assert her own independence by deciding for herself, without collaboration, the end of her therapy. Having considered these points, and wishing to create a balance between not disempowering her and leaving "the door open", I said, "Florence, you are right. I can see how you might feel that I don't understand your need for love. I just want to say that it is precisely because I have come to learn so much about you that I want us to deal with this together and decide what is best for you to do. Of course I will respect your final wish." Florence's defensiveness subsided and she apologised for "biting my head off". However, she decided that for now she no longer needed to see me, thanked me for all my help, and said that she appreciated my offer that she could contact me whenever she wished to resume her therapy.

It was six months later that I received a letter from Florence asking if she could see me again. It was a brief note saying that, although she and Chris were still seeing each other, they were having arguments because she would get very jealous and possessive and she was afraid of losing him. She also said that she wanted to see me before she was driven to "hit the bottle" again.

ABANDONMENT AND "GUIDED MOURNING"

Florence's letter was immensely gratifying because it conveyed her improved insight: she was able to recognise that her behaviour towards Chris was not helpful in maintaining their relationship; she was also able to foresee that her situation signalled a "danger spot" in relation to alcohol consumption; her initiative to get in touch with me not only confirmed her trust in our therapeutic relationship, but most of all it was the first indication that Florence was truly "growing" as a person and was prepared to take responsibility for her actions by making "adult" choices.

Meeting Florence again after six months was a very rewarding experience. Her decision to suspend her therapy had had a positive effect in that it provided her with an opportunity to rely on her own resources and had clearly increased her sense of self-efficacy. I reflected these feelings to her and she said, "I felt really bad after our last session. . . . I thought you might think I was selfish and ungrateful. Many times I felt like getting in touch, but was too proud to say you were right. Now I'm pleased that I tried to cope alone for a while and it made me realise so many things. . . . The most important of these, was to stop being a brat and to get a grip on my life, and I am now really honest when I say please help me to stop driving Chris away. . . . I also want to stop the urge to run towards alcohol for comfort."

With a "new lease of life", so to speak, to our therapeutic alliance, Florence and I were able to address her fear of abandonment in a constructive and collaborative manner, using schema-based approaches, joint sessions with Chris, and cognitive/behavioural experiments. The latter, inevitably, involved the issue of observing personal boundaries, eliciting emotional needs, and practising appropriate means of communicating these. At that stage of our work it became clear that there were times when Florence would become overwhelmed by emotions that she was unable to subject to some of the practical, self-coping strategies we discussed. For example, she felt very vulnerable at times when she perceived Chris to be drawing away from her, and even when she was able to realise that she had no grounds for such anxiety, her immediate thought was to turn to alcohol. Although she had not resorted to this, she said that she frequently "came very close" to doing so. I therefore decided to explore her willingness to be referred to a "mindfulness" group, which follows the principles of Linehan's work (see Chapter 12). After explaining to Florence that such a group is geared towards non-verbal means of deflecting anxiety and "letting go" of unhelpful thinking through the use of meditation techniques, her response was very positive and she agreed to try it out. Mindfulness training proved to be very successful for Florence and her commitment to the weekly group sessions, as well as daily training in meditation, provided her with a good technique for lowering "emotional noise" created in the present.

The impact of her unresolved grief about the loss of her father on her current situation was central to our work, and some individual sessions were devoted to bereavement work (Kubler-Ross, 1989). In particular, "guided mourning rituals" proved to be very effective in dealing with Florence's unprocessed loss that had remained frozen from the time of her father's death. She had, so far, avoided looking at any photographs of her father, and some of his items that she had kept in a box remained untouched from the moment they were put there. Together, we created a series of steps that involved looking at photographs, handling his possessions, and creating a shrine with flowers, which Florence could use as a focus of her guided mourning. These steps were by no means easy for her, but gradually they succeeded in freeing all the feelings she had bottled up, in particular her sadness, her anger, and the loss of her early happiness.

She volunteered that she wanted to travel back to the mainland to visit her father's grave, which is something she had never done from the time of his funeral. She also said that she wanted to take a letter she had written to him and place it at the grave because this would have more symbolic meaning. Her "goodbye" letter to him read as follows:

Dear Dad

It is only now that I've realised that I never let you go. I was so happy when you were around that I never wanted it to end. I think somewhere deep inside of me I hoped that you would somehow return to us and make everything better. I have also realised how angry I've been with you for leaving us, but because I loved you so much I couldn't accept my anger and took it out on myself, as well as others, instead. For a while I wanted to be like you and help our family stay united and happy, but another thing I now understand is how unrealistic that was. I was still growing and I needed love and attention, and instead I tried to be grown up before my time. Then the worst thing happened! Mum met a monster of a man who made all our lives miserable. . . . He did terrible things to me for which I've been so ashamed because I wanted to always be your eldest and special little girl. Instead, he made me feel dirty and I hated myself for it. The worst thing is that I took it out on poor Mum and blamed her for ruining our lives. The truth of it is that she was trying her best to create a family atmosphere for us, but she was his victim as well because he used to beat her black and blue. Fortunately, we managed to get rid of him before it was too late.

Dad, for a long time I felt like a failure who had made a terrible mess of her life and behaved like an angry spoiled brat, blaming everyone else, then feeling guilty and taking all the anger out on myself. I so much wanted you to be proud of me, and the more I failed the more I wanted to destroy myself. But now I want you to know that with help I am really beginning to feel normal—as though I'm finally growing up. I now know that I can't keep looking back, and I have to take my own responsibilities in life, as you used to. You were a wonderful man, always had a good word for people, however bad they were. You were loving and fair, and did your best to teach us right from wrong. It is these things which I must now cherish and thank you for having given me, and use them wisely! I'm even beginning to realise that I have that wicked sense of humour of yours and I know that you would be proud of me no matter what. I hope they are looking after you well up there, otherwise they'll have me to contend with!

Love you lots, always!

Goodbye and rest in peace

Florence

Florence read out her letter to me prior to going on her pilgrimage trip and it was a very emotional and significant stage of the therapy for both of us, after which we remained in reflective silence for some time. Her words, in my opinion, succinctly encapsulated the current location of Florence's journey toward freedom and growth, better than any learned formulation.

FINAL CHALLENGE: SEXUAL ABUSE RESOLUTION

On Florence's return from her very important trip, we had a review session in order to evaluate her progress and address her remaining needs. The moment she entered the room I could detect that some very significant changes in her had taken place. Once again, it was that very satisfying and familiar intuitive feeling of knowing that a survivor had turned a very important corner. She looked relaxed, confident, and for the first time exuded a sense of peace as though a very heavy burden had been lifted. She started the session by saying, "I feel as though I am finally in charge of my life. Going to say goodbye to Dad was not easy but now I feel at peace with myself. All of the goals I set myself so long ago seem to be coming together. I went to see my mother of course, and we had a very emotional reunion. In fact all of the family came over and it felt wonderful to see them again . . . it was as though we were starting over." After I acknowledged that, indeed, she seemed very well and happy and that I was very pleased, Florence looked at me and said, "There is only one small shadow on the horizon. . . . I don't want to keep thinking of "him", and feel bad about what he did to me. I know now that I wasn't to blame, but I can't help feeling disgusted whenever I remember what he used to say and do."

On further exploration of these feelings, Florence said that mostly she did not think of the abuse, and it was only when she was intimate with Chris that she would feel inhibited and unable to be spontaneous. At this point, she connected with the fact that she used to use alcohol in her previous relationships in order to be able to "perform", because she thought that this was what the men expected from her. Now that she was sober, she found it hard to relax and assumed that any sexual act she became involved with would define her as a "loose" woman. That is not to say that she did not enjoy sex, but that she had come to associate sexual behaviour with depravity. It was when we identified the consequences that these beliefs had on her self-image as well as her relationship, that the final stages of the therapy were defined, namely in terms of her self-esteem and the quality of her relationship with Chris.

With an increasingly solid new foundation that Florence had worked very hard to achieve, resolving the effects of the sexual abuse did not prove to be very difficult. Indeed, issues of powerlessness and control were relatively minor as compared with the enduring and unhelpful personal statements Florence had nurtured over the years. In wanting to preserve her relationship with Chris, her belief had dramatically shifted from once believing that she had to be sexually available to a man in order to keep him, to now assuming that she had to be almost chaste for Chris to perceive her as a worthy partner. Our work, therefore, focused mainly on challenging the usefulness of her assumptions in the light of the fact that she was now learning to adopt more balanced "schemas", or patterns with which to manage her life. Including Chris in our sessions was particularly helpful to Florence, because hearing his views within a "non-threatening" and objective context allowed her to question the validity of her beliefs and also appreciate his.

CONCLUDING SESSIONS: INDEPENDENCE AND GROWTH

It was nearly four years from the time I first met Florence to when her therapy came to an end (including the periodic follow-ups). I was privileged indeed to be party to the growth of this initially very unhappy and disturbed young woman, who gradually emerged as a complete being who was able to make informed choices about her life.

The ups and downs of our therapeutic alliance provided me with opportunities for my own development, both professional and personal. I was made acutely aware that it is all too easy to blame the patient when things are not going smoothly by assuming that they are either too disturbed to benefit from therapy, or that they are simply "not ready" for it. By being prepared to make it my responsibility whether Florence engaged with me or not, I was able to stretch my clinical and personal resources in my duty to do all I could to provide her with a congruent, safe, and empathic base from which to address her distress. My role as limited parent was particularly challenged when working with Florence, and she too found my (at times necessary but constructive) confrontations quite difficult, but she was to tell me later, "I'm so grateful for all the times when you didn't let me get away with my unreasonable behaviour. . . . It made me realise how much I'd missed out on guidance and a firm hand."

Florence's personal growth can best be understood in terms of her changing attitudes and beliefs in three areas: herself; other people; and the world in general. Her initial self-chastisement, as well as raging anger towards the family whom she felt had let her down, gave way to insightful understanding about the complexities of life where blame cannot be a substitute for taking personal responsibility. Having her pain and abuse validated allowed Florence to start literally growing emotionally and eventually achieving her potential as an adult. More crucially, at about three-quarters of the way into her therapy, she started showing those very familiar signs of being able to be empathic towards other people. In my experience, survivors, as well as other clients who have suffered varying types of abuse, are so preoccupied by their own pain and what they perceive to be the injustice of it, that they do not possess the capacity to be aware of and empathic of other people's life struggles. Florence's growing self-worth and understanding of the world's inevitable injustice, but also potential for joy and success, extended her horizons in both the interpersonal and practical dimensions.

Towards the end of her therapy she expressed some sentiments that I have often heard from other survivors and which are very powerful in describing their new found freedom. She said, "There is something very exciting, but also very frightening about how I feel now. It is as though I am a new person who can have a fresh start to life and can be like everyone else. The scary thing is that now I know that I will never be able to use all of my old excuses and do the things I used to do because I can see clearly what will happen if I do. . . . It is a bit daunting being a grown up, but I'm grateful that I'm here."

Addressing her last observation constituted the closing sessions towards Florence's independence from therapy. As we tackled the various aspects of being an adult that Florence found daunting, her realisation that she was now well equipped for the remaining journey of her life afforded her a further insight. The latter referred to her appreciation that life can be hard and that it would be unrealistic for her to expect that all would be plain sailing from now on. What was different now was that she had become, in her own words, "the master of my ship". This allowed me to quote to her a saying I once heard that "Life is not a pleasure cruise, but a journey in uncharted waters, where being in charge of the ship is what sees us through the difficulties". Our ability to share this "wisdom" in a relatively light-hearted manner while understanding its meaning, and without my fearing that Florence would be overwhelmed and invalidated, was a reassuring signal of her readiness to leave the therapy.

In the periodic follow-up sessions prior to final termination of our therapy, Florence and I would share various anecdotes, and I frequently commented on how funny she was and that I looked forward to seeing her as she made me laugh. Her humour had progressed from the cynical to the witty, and I was particularly amused when on our last day she said, "Making you laugh was the least I could do after all you've done for me. Now, don't tell me that you'll miss me and that you can't survive without my jokes, because it's tough . . . after all the bird must fly the nest!" She was a little tearful when she was saying this, and it was her way of showing me she was being brave and she no longer needed her safety net.

Florence eventually left the island and returned to the mainland to be near her family. She sent me the occasional postcard, and, about a year and a half after I had last seen her, she telephoned me to say that she had married Chris and was expecting their first child. This was the last ever contact I had from her and her parting comments were: "Remember that business about the cruise ship you were going on about? Well, I can tell you that it has indeed not been plain sailing all the way, but I'm really getting the hang of being the captain. . . . Well, I have to, there will be a brat on board soon!"

Chapter 12

The case studies: Closing remarks

Florence's progress in therapy completes the case studies of survivors of childhood sexual abuse I chose in order to illustrate the many facets of their troubled lives, and the implementation of an integrated working model in order to facilitate the resolution of the long-term effects of their experience. At initial presentation, Florence's personal resources were at a level that did not enable her to cope with life's daily demands, or to regulate her relationships in the general, family, and intimate domain in an adaptive manner. The parameters of my conceptualisation of her difficulties within an Axis II diagnosis of borderline personality disorder, underpinned by the experience of loss, sexual abuse, and disrupted family dynamics, acted as my own crucial guide towards establishing and maintaining our therapeutic relationship and remaining vigilant to the inevitable see-sawing between engagement and ruptures (Silk et al, 1997). A particular challenge was the need for careful integration and blending of a variety of techniques that would address Florence's difficulties, while at the same time not losing sight of her need for validation, guidance, and the opportunity to learn to trust.

Shortly after the traumatic loss of her father, Florence and her siblings were introduced to a man who, for want of a better description, was to wage a campaign of terror characterised by verbal, sexual, and physical violence. The family's previous peaceful equilibrium having been brutally disturbed, set off a chain of events that Florence, her siblings, and her mother were at a loss to know how to reinstate. More crucially, Florence's adaptation in this atmosphere of perpetual "emotional noise" was to assume responsibility in her attempt to maintain a semblance of the family togetherness she had previously experienced. The long-term result was that this "noise" failed to abate, either because she unwittingly recreated similar situations with her sexual partners, or because inability to trust herself and others resulted in emotional conflicts or self-destructive acts.

With respect to the above, I was hugely inspired by the work of Linehan (1993, 1998), which adopts a "dialectical" approach in the treatment of personality disorder. While schema-focused work helped Florence and I to identify and then work through the specific unhelpful patterns or "stencils" that regulated her world, the incorporation of "mindfulness" as a here and now strategy that could help her reduce emotional tension proved to be a successful adjunct (see Kabat-Zinn, 1990). Linehan's work astutely combines behavioural skills with Zen Buddhist meditation in an attempt at increasing the personal effectiveness and empowerment of clients who have experienced abusive upbringings, and particularly in clients with BPD. This approach has also recently received particular attention for its potential towards reducing relapse in depression (Teasdale, 2000).

A further point that merits highlighting concerns Florence's disclosure of her abuse to her mother. Reactions of mothers to their daughters' disclosures will be addressed in Chapter 13, but suffice it to say that for Florence, her mother's validation of her abuse and the fact that she was prepared to take steps to remove her husband from the family home, had far-reaching implications for their long-term relationship, and for Florence's self-esteem (Crawford, 1999; Lange et al, 1999; Morrow and Sorell, 1989). Indeed, the potential for resolution of Florence's complex cluster of difficulties was greatly enhanced by two main factors: her experience of a loving and stable base up to the age of nine; and the continuing bond with her mother and the latter's positive reaction to the disclosure of her daughter's abuse.

As with Victoria and Rose, Florence's story once again brings to attention the sharp relevance of the developmental perspective. In addition, their experience, as well as that of other survivors, points to the dearth of current knowledge about the specific parameters of family functioning and their relationship to long-term adjustment of survivors of sexual abuse (Weissmann-Wind and Silvern, 1994; Faust et al, 1995). The chapter that follows will focus on these issues as well as the impact on families following disclosure of sexual abuse.

I am well aware that for obvious reasons it was not possible to include every single facet of the experience of sexual abuse in the case studies that have been presented. I am confident, however, that I have taken great care to portray the central recurring themes in the presentation of survivors, as well as the common long-term effects that they experience. It is hoped, therefore, that the case studies will have inspired the reader, and that the conceptualisations and techniques discussed will offer valuable guidance.

It is important that I reiterate the fact that while the length of interventions I have just presented ranged from one to four years, there is great variability in duration of therapy for survivors of sexual abuse. In my own experience over the past decade, the number of sessions with survivors who completed their therapy has ranged from as little as a handful of sessions to as many as eighty; these have been spread over a few weeks in the first instance and up to five years in the second, with great variability in between, depending on the requirements of a particular survivor.

Although a number of therapeutic techniques have been mentioned, I have anticipated that the issue of group therapy, or lack of it, might be queried. Over the course of my work on the island, I have extensively addressed the possibility of setting up a therapeutic group and/or indeed a support group for survivors. The response was not favourable as survivors have repeatedly expressed their wish for anonymity within a community the size of which renders it difficult to maintain. I have of course understood and respected this, but feel fortunate to be able to gain access for my patients to closed "mindfulness" meditation groups (see Linehan in the above discussion), which are set up by an experienced group leader and colleague who, as well as being a psychologist, has the added advantage of being an ordained lay Zen Buddhist monk. Her training groups have provided an invaluable adjunct to therapy for those survivors who are troubled by intense emotions, which are not sufficiently regulated by cognitive/behavioural or schema-based work alone.

Last but by no means least, I should point out that while I have provided three illustrations of how memories of sexual abuse are dealt with, in terms of varying degrees of intrusiveness, it is in Chapter 14 that I address the issue of "recovered" memories in relation to their purpose in the thera-peutic context, and the situations where encouraging their recollection is contra-indicated.

Part IV

The families, disclosure, and the role of the mother

Chapter 13

Survivors' families and the impact of disclosure

In Chapter 5 several references were made to the relevance and importance of family dynamics as mediators of long-term effects experienced by survivors of child sexual abuse (CSA). Moreover, the reader may also recall that when describing the particular difficulties reported by survivors who were coping "very badly" or "badly" at initial presentation for therapy, I presented a crude classification of the types of family environment these survivors described. In this chapter, I take up these classifications and discuss them in terms of two issues: first, I attempt to offer conceptualisations that I believe to be most relevant to the types of family background described by the survivors whom I have treated; and, secondly, I discuss the process of disclosure of CSA (when this occurs) by survivors and the perceived impact this had on all of those involved. Based on survivors' subjective reports, the role of the mother assumes particular importance when addressing these issues. A further subjective report of note concerns the relationship of perpetrators to survivors. In view of the fact that the majority of survivors whom I have seen reported intrafamilial CSA and, in particular, by a father or substitute father figure, and also the fact that most studies in this area are based on incest abuse (e.g. Armstrong, 1978; LaBarbera et al, 1980; Herman, 1981; Dadds et al, 1991; Lipovsky et al, 1992; Faust et al, 1995; Crawford, 1999; Melchert, 2000; Marshall et al, 2000), the discussion that follows focuses mainly on intrafamilial CSA.

I would contend that any attempts by us as professionals or even researchers to conceptualise the internal workings of a family ultimately can only be subjective and/or theoretical, although generalisations abound. This observation is the more pertinent in the context of CSA, which continues to be an area of enormous complexity and challenge due to the profoundly private nature of family structure in general, and the endemic rule of secrecy (and also coercion) that governs abusive families in particular. Even when families are subjected to the scrutiny of intervening or treating professionals, most of us would agree that what we observe might be only the tip of a very large iceberg. What happens behind closed doors is experienced in its relative entirety only by the cohabitants of the family domain, whose members can choose what and what not to reveal to the outside world, or indeed, to each other. It is precisely this latter observation that many survivors repeatedly make when they vent their frustration and disappointment that their suffering as children was either not noticed, or that when it was, nothing happened to stop it. This issue will be discussed further in the closing chapter of this book, but for the moment I would like to discuss the conceptual frameworks that I have found to be of relevance when trying to understand survivors' descriptions of their families during the course of their therapy.

SURVIVORS' FAMILIES AND RELEVANT CONCEPTUALISATIONS

The "chaotic" and "unstable" family environments which survivors described were characterised by dysfunction in terms of inadequate parenting and abdication of responsibilities; poor parental personal resources and dependency; couple dissatisfaction and unstable power dynamics; and loss of one or both parental figures. The sexual abuse experienced by survivors in this type of family was, in the majority of cases, intrafamilial, and it was not uncommon for them to have also been abused by outsiders. It was also not uncommon for them to have been verbally and/or physically abused, and to have experienced physical and emotional neglect. Frequently, particularly if they were the elder sibling, they would have taken responsibility for younger members of the family. Referring to Winnicott's assertion that "Home is where we start from", and that "the home is the parents', not the child's responsibility" (Winnicott, 1986, p.124), these environments contravened almost all of the requirements that can facilitate a child's transition and adaptation into adult society.

The "incongruous" type of family described by survivors, while appearing for all intents and purposes to function well, was perceived by them as being inconsistent and living a life that was rife with double standards. Such families appear to adopt a strict moral code and it is not unusual for them to be church devotees. The most pertinent double standard reported by survivors was their parents' vehement verbal chastisement of what they considered to be debauched sexual behaviour, while the survivors themselves were being subjected to unjust sexual insults, improper personal boundaries and, of course, abuse. In these families the power was usually firmly held by one of the parents, the other of whom would abdicate most responsibilities and would tend to be absent as a consistent caregiver. What appears to be particularly characteristic of these families is their insularity from the outside world, which of course renders detection of the abuse, let alone help, almost impossible. While CSA was almost always incestuous in such families, it was also the case, in some instances, that outside family members were also involved.

While CSA may not be automatically assumed to occur in all chaotic, unstable, and incongruous environments, the latter, nevertheless, may provide the necessary conditions for it to occur; this will be discussed a little later. The "emotionally inhibited" type of environment I described in Chapter 5 differs significantly from the three types mentioned above, as it is the type of "ordinary" family that docs not attract particular social attention. Here it is more difficult to explore antecedents for CSA and it is only during closer scrutiny, particularly based on survivors' verbal reports, that one can appreciate their lack of close emotional parental attachments, and the isolation they experienced, both prior to as well as following their sexual abuse. Interestingly, however, it is mostly within these families that validation of the abuse, when disclosure occurred, was more likely to be forthcoming, as well as a genuine willingness to provide help and support. The sexual abuse was more likely to be perpetrated by friends or close relatives, not usually inhabiting the family home.

A number of hypotheses have been discussed in order to explain the antecedents of CSA (Courtois, 1988; Edwards and Alexander, 1992; Kirschner et al, 1993; Faust et al, 1995). Bearing in mind, however, that what is discussed here refers directly to the survivors' subjective reports, I was struck by the universal idealisation of the "mother" as the ultimate figure who acts as a repository in which most of the intense and ambivalent emotions about childhood experience is stored. Indeed, so significant a role did the mother appear to assume for most of the survivors I have seen to date, that the nearest approximation to this significance I was able to find was in Bowlby's theory of attachment and loss (Bowlby, 1973, 1980, 1988), which stipulates not only that a child requires a stable and secure base from which to explore his/her environment effectively, but that while secure attachment with both parents predicts optimal outcome in adult social and relationship adjustment, infant–mother attachment is superior to infant–father attachment in predicting such outcome. Combining these arguments, Alexander's (1992) examination of the antecedents of CSA using attachment theory succeeds, at least partly in my opinion, because not only does it take into account both mother and father figures but, more crucially, it highlights the importance of taking into consideration the interactions between the whole family when looking at the onset of CSA. The author quotes Sroufe et al (1985) as saying: "Viewing the family as a system . . . implies interconnections among relationships; that is, one relationship has implications for other relationships within the system" (p. 317).

Alexander's conceptualisation

Alexander's conceptualisation rests on the initial premise that sexual abuse is frequently linked to the intergenerational transmission of insecure attachment, whether or not there is intergenerational abuse. Furthermore, her theory posits that the onset of CSA is preceded by insecure attachment in the parent, and she employs three types of such attachment: role reversal/parentification; fear; and rejection. The first is supported by earlier empirical evidence (Levang, 1989) and is described as the experience whereby the child is parentified to the extent that he/she is abused by a parent whose sense of entitlement creates in him/her the expectation that the child should meet his/her sexual and emotional needs. The conditions for CSA to occur are further reinforced by the inability of the non-abusing parent, who may themselves have been parentified in their childhood, to attend to their child's emotional needs. Moreover, the non-abusing parent (almost always the mother in the case of the survivors I have seen) may be lacking in the appropriate emotional and/or cognitive resources to be able to stop the abuse from occurring. Indeed, the majority of survivors whom I saw held a strong belief that their mothers were in some way aware of the abuse and held deep resentment that they were unable to stop it. What angered them further was their constant concern over younger siblings whom they felt an obligation to protect, leading them to allow the abuse to continue in the hope that it would save the younger ones from such an experience. This scenario was particularly expressed in survivors who described chaotic, unstable, and incongruous family environments.

The second family antecedent to CSA explored by Alexander refers to disorganised attachment based on parental unresolved trauma and fear. This situation is certainly frequently found in the chaotic type of environments, which are characterised by numerous problems involving substance abuse, physical abuse, and indiscriminate sexual behaviour. Here, the abusing parents' attempts to deal with their disorganised attachment based on fear of abandonment and history of CSA through dissociation and substance abuse, is argued to lead to a reduction in impulse control. On the other hand, the non-abusing parent who may themselves have experienced a similar childhood, may find themselves in a situation whereby their own fear of abandonment and dissolution of the family within an all too familiar scenario may reinforce their own helplessness and lack of resources to defend the child. Moreover, the mother (as the most frequent non-abusing parent in the current survivors) may consciously or unconsciously fail to see evidence for the abuse, and may indeed, protest its non-existence when faced with her child's disclosure. This issue will be addressed further when I discuss the process of disclosure later in this chapter.

Finally, insecure attachment modulated by rejection is the final antecedent to CSA examined by Alexander (1992). This theme has been previously discussed by Zeanah and Zeanah (1989), and describes a situation whereby avoidant attachment in the child due to rejection makes the latter feel unwanted and unloved, while the avoidant, or absent parent tends to be unavailable, psychologically and/or physically. Based on survivors' reports, this situation best typifies the "incongruous" type of family described earlier, and occasionally the "emotionally inhibited" one. Alexander's critique concerns itself mostly with the scenario whereby the avoidant authoritarian father is usually the perpetrator of the child's abuse, due to his belief that his children as well as his spouse are his property, while the mother, as the subjugated wife, is incapable of making herself available to her children. This is argued to be due to her inevitable physical absence as a result of an overload of responsibilities within the home and also outside it, and her emotional unavailability due to her own neglect, depression, or other psychological difficulties. The point is made that the child who develops avoidant attachment in this situation, due to rejection, runs not only the risk of becoming vulnerable to other types of incestuous abuse, but is also unlikely to be able to defend itself against the abuse, and even less likely to seek help from others.

While I have certainly heard countless survivors describe their feelings of rejection within an atmosphere of alienation from both parents, it has frequently been the case that it was the mother who was the strict authoritarian household figure, and the father or father figure who was subjugated, as well as being the perpetrator of the abuse. In such a scenario, it is reasonable to assume that both rejection and role reversal are important family dynamics within the context of CSA. Indeed, taking survivors' histories as a whole, it is also reasonable to assume that one or more of the three types of insecure attachments described are playing an important role in the emergence and maintenance of CSA.

Alexander's theory has certainly been very useful as well as pertinent when attempting to understand survivors' personal histories. Indeed, it was my primary concern that I discuss the conceptualisation of attachment because I have found it to be the one that most approximated the survivors' experience of their childhood. I am only too aware, however, that attachment and systems theories of family functioning have received ample criticism (e.g. Birns and Meyer, 1993; Crawford, 1999) in an attempt to exonerate mothers from the butt of patriarchal or unfounded attack. It is hoped, however, that the reader will appreciate that I am validating the survivors by presenting their accounts, and also that I have attempted to create a balance between survivors' perceptions and the dynamics of the family as a whole. More crucially, it is my opinion that this discussion would be incomplete, and also irresponsible, if two further important factors where omitted: the psychology of child sex offenders; and the role of society. The degree to which I consider these issues to be important is such that I have accorded them particular attention in the final chapter of this book. Suffice it to say, that the uncontrolled impulses of child sex offenders, as a result of childhood or adolescent conditioning variables, as well as genetic and personality factors, irrespective of the theoretical frameworks discussed in relation to antecedents of CSA, may have, arguably, singular significance in the onset and perpetuation of CSA.

I accord equal importance to the role that all of us, in our society, have in terms of taking a degree of responsibility towards the well-being of children. It is easy to be distanced and smug and accord blame or point the finger at dysfunctional families and assume that if only they were able to change, or become educated, or allow us to help them, then abuse would not occur; I believe this to be a very short-sighted approach. In fact, I would further suggest that there is no such thing as the "ideal family", and that while in principle we can all strive towards being the type of parents who will provide the best possible start for our children, we can all fall from the pedestal. I, personally, believe that family functioning is a dimension within which any of us may be striving to reach the edge of ideal parenthood. The point is made, however, that there are numerous individual, sociobiological and cultural factors that can either facilitate or hinder this process. Furthermore, the whole issue of sexual abuse is still one that arouses in society the types of responses—namely distaste and horror—which do not allow for greater knowledgeable awareness of the issue and deter us from becoming purposefully engaged in child protection.

DISCLOSURE AND ROLE OF THE MOTHER

As in the previous section, some of the issues that will be discussed here may be of a somewhat sensitive nature. Once again, my purpose is to convey to the reader the types of experience survivors related on the occasions when they disclosed their abuse to their families. I considered this to be important, particularly in view of the fact that I was unable to find specific empirical work that has sought to examine the experience of adult survivors following their disclosure of abuse. Indeed, overall, there is little empirical work about the impact child disclosure of CSA can have on families (e.g. Davies, 1995; Nagel et al, 1997), or retrospective studies involving the adult survivors who have made such disclosures (e.g. Finkelhor, 1979; Bagley and Ramsay, 1986; Everill and Waller, 1995; Ussher and Dewberry, 1995).

Of the 180 survivors discussed in this book, about half had disclosed the abuse to their families, and this occurred mostly when they were adults, or during middle or late adolescence. Indeed, a few of these disclosures occurred during the course of their therapy. Although the remainder did not wish to make either formal or informal disclosures and sought alternative ways of confronting their experience of abuse, a number of the women made a few interesting observations. For example, many women recalled, as children, telling their parents and, in particular, their mothers, that they did not wish to visit their grandparents or that they hated being left alone in the house with elder brothers, father figures, or neighbours, but the situation was never systematically explored further with them. Although they also recalled not being able to make concrete accusations, they did remember being unhappy and "playing up" to the extent that they were viewed as spoilt and disruptive, and typically being told not to make a fuss or be so ungrateful, because after all, "Uncle Harry is such a nice, generous man!" More tragically, a small number of survivors recalled that despite being seen by medical and/or child guidance professionals due to chronic urinary infections and other signs of abuse, as well as behavioural problems, no action was taken towards further investigation.

Patterns of disclosure and perceived impact

I will illustrate survivors' experience of disclosure during adulthood in terms of two extreme parental reactions. The first represents the worst outcome following disclosure and is characterised by intense family disruption that has serious consequences for all those involved, and especially for the survivor. In such cases, there is usually the added stress and apprehension of making formal complaints, which may or may not lead to the arrest of the perpetrator, and of course the uncertainty that such procedures will culminate in convicting the latter. In my experience, I have found no typical antecedents to making the disclosure, although there are a number of precipitating factors. Pre-therapy—i.e. when survivors have already made the disclosure—the psychological and emotional consequences for them can be particularly severe because they are not benefiting from appropriate guidance and support. Indeed, it is not unusual for survivors to seek professional help after they have initiated their disclosure, which may have been instigated for a number of reasons: there may be concern about the survivor's children or the children of the perpetrator, or any vulnerable children known to the survivor and also the perpetrator; a further reason may be the accumulation of psychological distress and anger, with an intense feeling of injustice about perceiving oneself to be suffering and also to be affecting the lives of loved ones, while the perpetrator is not brought to account for his actions. There is also frequently the situation whereby one of a group of siblings and/or friends initiates the disclosure of her abuse to a sister or close friend. In many cases, such disclosures result in no more than a welcome alleviation of the burden of holding on to a lifelong secret, as it is usually met by empathy, concern, and support. It can also be the case, however, that the disclosure may set off a crisis and a chain of events not foreseen by the survivor. For example, the other sibling or friend may disclose that she too was abused by the same perpetrator, which culminates in the disclosure of all parties to their families, frequently progressing to making formal statements to the police. A further unexpected result of such disclosure is that the non-abused sibling, relative, or friend, on receiving the news, experiences a conflict between offering support and split loyalties that may culminate in denial of the survivor's confession, and worst still, she/he closes ranks with the perpetrator and his supporters.

Due to these very complex possible ramifications, I would always advocate that any type of disclosure by a survivor is best done with the help of an experienced professional in the field of CSA. There is nothing worse for a survivor than to feel further disempowered and isolated from the family network, not to mention the trauma of making detailed police statements, without appropriate guidance and support. The greatest source of distress in these situations, however, is the survivors' experience of parental denial, anger, and rejection of them as the responsible instigators of family strife. Mothers, in particular, have been described in such scenarios by the survivor as being, at best ambivalent about the news that their daughter was abused as a child, and at worst as accusing them of fabricating malicious lies in order to disrupt the family, typically saying: "You must really hate me . . . whatever have I done to deserve such treatment?" Further, the survivor may be blamed for causing the breakdown of the mother's relationship with her partner as well as creating gossip and isolation from family and acquaintances. A number of survivors who sought help following their disclosure to their mothers were particularly distraught about the fact that, while in the initial stages of the secret "coming out" they received appropriate support from her which was reinforced by banishing the perpetrator, when the perpetrator happened to be the mother's partner the latter was reinstated in the marital home within months of the expulsion, even in cases where court proceedings culminated in a conviction.

The attention given to mothers in these extreme negative response examples following the disclosure of CSA, directly reflects the purpose and intensity with which the survivors chose to relate their experience. Birns and Meyer (1993) take issue with focusing on mothers because they consider them to be victims of a patriarchal system that seeks to oppress all women, and that attributing blame to them for their daughter's abuse succeeds only in adding further credence to such a system. I would argue, however, that their stance is more theoretical and political than one borne out of clinical experience. While there may a great deal of truth in their critique, led by the experiences of the women whom I have treated I prefer to view the issue of mothers from a completely different perspective. I have been made rudely aware of the paramount importance that mothers have, not only for survivors of CSA but also for all the women whom I have seen to date. More crucially, this importance appears to involve no cultural, ethnic, or geographical distinctions. The idealisation of the mother figure as the primary protector and nurturer, and as the person who has the capacity to heal all ills, has been presented by survivors with emphatic alacrity. To enter into a theoretical discussion about this state of affairs and the reasons that conspire to prevent mothers from fulfilling such awesome expectations, would require a tome in itself; for an elaborate critique on motherhood, the interested reader is referred to the work of Estelle Welldon (1988).

Here, I wish to convey the fact that for survivors of CSA the degree of power of validation and positive response from their mothers following disclosure appears to be significantly greater than the trauma of the abuse itself. I have not encountered such strength of feeling towards fathers who have either denied or validated the abuse of their daughters. It is precisely because of this potentially vital link in the recovery of survivors that I, as a therapist, would fail in my role and duty if I were to politicise the aims of the therapy by embarking on an educational trail of gender roles in society. Not only would I fail in empathising with the pain of survivors, but would also fail in validating their experience and coming to terms with their grief. Ironically, when survivors have attained the level of independence and growth which I have illustrated in the previous chapters, they are able to recognise that their mothers were fallible human beings who were subject to the types of unhelpful and destructive patterns that they themselves experienced. It is as though the umbilical cord has been finally severed and they can emerge as whole and independent human beings.

The power of maternal capacity towards healing is best illustrated in the cases when disclosure of CSA was met with a positive response. Here, three general scenarios were described, and it may be coincidental that in all of them, professional intervention was already in place. The first situation was that of survivors who expressed a concern that their therapy would be incomplete unless they found the courage to confront their abuser. This issue was usually addressed with lengthy discussion about all the possible outcomes of such confrontation, the survivors' emotional resources, and rehearsal of the means by which to undertake such action in a way that would be least likely to lead to further distress. Some survivors chose to disclose the abuse to their mothers, in the first instance. Indeed, on a number of occasions, the survivors suggested disclosing the abuse during their therapy session with their mothers present. The frequency of such scenarios was relatively small, but when it occurred and succeeded (i.e. in terms of the mothers' positive response), the progress and outcome of therapy was substantially enhanced. Indeed, it was not unusual for the therapy to reach its conclusion, with the survivor perceiving that the resolution of their painful experience had been achieved. Their recovery in these situations was particularly speeded by their mothers' willingness and courage to stand by their daughters and banish the abuser from their lives, irrespective of whether they were their partners, extended family members, or friends. For survivors, this represented the ultimate validation of their experience and struggle towards health.

In the second scenario, when survivors opted for confronting their abuser on their own, a great deal of preparation took place in terms of the issues that I highlighted earlier. This, in my experience, constituted the most "risky" and potentially dangerous means of disclosure in survivors' perception. I sincerely admire and respect the courage of the women who chose this route, which they viewed as the only significant means of banishing the nightmares of their past. It must be said, that this type of disclosure occurred infrequently, but encouragingly for the survivors involved, it was a highly positive and satisfying experience. For them, it represented the ultimate means of regaining power over their lives, because the perpetrators acknowledged the abuse and indeed, in some cases, asked for forgiveness. Once again, the role of the mother proved to be of great significance when the latter, although usually shocked (particularly if the abuser was her partner, son, or father), provided appropriate support and allowed her daughter to express her wishes regarding further action. Similarly to the previous pattern of disclosure, these cases constituted the final and, possibly, the most significant link in the conclusion of survivors' therapy.

The third pattern of disclosure involved both parents' immediate validation and support following the disclosure of their daughter's abuse. This was likely to be the outcome when disclosure was concerned with extra-familial abuse or when the perpetrator, although a close relative, was not usually resident in the family home. Here, the survivor was likely to be in mid or late adolescence, and to be already receiving professional help due to psychological problems, particularly eating disorders and suicidal behaviour. The initial disclosure was usually made to one of the caring professionals who subsequently facilitated the "opening up of the secret". It is not unusual for older adolescents to be subsequently referred for individual therapy.

In instances when I have been involved with such survivors, it was an exceptional situation when both parents maintained an active, consistent, and participatory role during the therapeutic process. This background provided the best possible outcome for individual therapy, particularly when there was good communication between all of the professionals involved. Interestingly, even here, it was mainly at the mothers' initiative that communication was ensured, and when meeting with them (with survivors' consent) I was able to gain a measure of their deep concern and willingness to be guided towards the well-being of their daughters.

SUMMARY AND CONCLUSIONS

This chapter discussed the types of family background that survivors described, the reasons for their disclosure of CSA (when this occurred), the various patterns of such disclosure, and the role of the mother. I have sought to convey, primarily, the experience of survivors whom I have treated, and while all of the issues mentioned are argued to be significant variables in the experience and resolution of CSA, I have noted a dearth of well-controlled studies concerning them. Although there is a substantial amount of clinical and theoretical work concerning the families of survivors of CSA, it remains unclear whether we have a coherent picture of ante-cedents most likely to facilitate such abuse. While I have recognised the difficulties inherent in conducting such studies, the latter are, nevertheless, urgently needed.

In addition, there is an urgent need for work in the area of patterns of disclosure in adulthood, and the role of parents, extended family, and, more crucially, mothers, when disclosure of CSA occurs. My therapeutic experi-ence leads me to believe that the fear and apprehension of disclosure is acute and that when this happens, it can either significantly hinder, or substantially enhance the course of recovery, depending on the perceived reactions of the recipients of the news.

Finally, I stressed the point that viewing the family as the sole and primary factor in the incidence of CSA is not only short-sighted, but also dangerous. I brought attention to paedophilia as being, arguably, the most significant factor in the perpetuation of CSA, and propose to discuss this issue in the final chapter of this book. In addition, I stressed the importance of the role of society in its efforts to make concerted efforts in assuming a responsible and proactive stance towards child protection. This issue is also discussed in Chapter 15.[1]

Part V

Further considerations

Chapter 14

The "recovered/false" memory debate

This brief chapter has been included for the sake of completeness. Controversial as it might sound, while I have followed the debate with keen academic interest and have accorded its concerns appropriate caution, I have found the issues regarding recovered and false memories to be of little or no direct relevance to my own clinical involvement with survivors of sexual abuse, and I shall be discussing the reasons for this a little later. In the first instance, I will present a summary of the background to the debate and of the current state of affairs.

BACKGROUND

The phrases "recovered memories" and "false memory syndrome" assumed particular importance in the early 1990s, and arguably more so in the USA, when a backlash involving the legal system and families who alleged to being falsely accused by their grown-up children of sexually abusing them during their childhood began to emerge. The notion of "therapy" that "uncovers" abuse became in some circles the *bête noire*, encompassing at worst aberrant and unethical professional behaviour, and at best unreliable and ill-informed practice. Two influential bodies that emerged as a result of this situation were the False Memory Syndrome Foundation (FMSF), which was formed in Philadelphia in 1992, and the British False Memory Society (BFMS) in the United Kingdom, which came together in 1993.

Initially, much of the debate concerning the authenticity of disclosures of CSA took place in the public arena. One side of the camp consisted of people who claimed to have recovered traumatic memories of abuse, as well as therapists who reported to have observed this phenomenon in their consulting rooms. The other side of the debate included those who were accused of perpetrating the abuse, and some researchers who purported that the bizarre content of recovered memories, and the dubious nature of certain therapeutic techniques such as hypnosis and regression, invalidated such claims. The degree of concern in both camps—i.e. that, on the one hand, incidents of genuine abuse would be refuted, while on the other, innocent people would be falsely accused—prompted British, Australian, and American psychologists to form working parties in order to review both empirical and therapeutic aspects of these issues. In particular, in 1995 members of the British Psychological Society's working party on recovered memories carried out a national survey (Andrews et al, 1995). Over 4,000 questionnaires were sent to members of relevant divisions within the Society, with the aim of attempting to address issues relating to the extent to which Society practitioners encounter clients who recover memories while in their care; the belief of practitioners regarding the accuracy of such memories; and the extent to which memories are recovered prior to entering therapy and whether these memories are only specific to CSA. The results of this survey are discussed in the May 1995 edition of the *Psychologist*. Suffice it to say that the overall conclusions were that memory recovery is a robust and frequent phenomenon that is not limited to CSA, nor to survivors of CSA. More crucially, it was suggested that the recovery of memory cannot be solely attributed to untrained therapists and/or thera-peutic techniques, and that the use of hypnotic regression was a rare occurrence among the highly trained survey respondents. The closing remarks of this survey referred to the fact that there was an urgent need for research into the process, context, and validity of recovered memories. Interestingly, the latter conclusion was also reached in 1994 by the con-tributions of cognitive researchers and therapists in two journal issues, *Applied Cognitive Psychology* and *Consciousness and Cognition*, which were solely devoted to the topic.

In 1995, Withers and Mitchell raised a very important issue. They were concerned that scepticism towards accounts of CSA by the BFMS lobby could potentially have damaging effects on the large number of genuine survivors. The authors also argued that while they had sympathy for inno-cent alleged perpetrators of abuse, they were anxious that the questioning of the prevalence of CSA was reminiscent of Freud's seduction theory and his refutation of his previously held belief that several of his female patients had experienced traumas of a sexual nature. Indeed, Masson (1989) pro-posed that Freud's refutation of his original theory was in response to the criticisms of colleagues which led to a revised theory stating that claims of sexual abuse by fathers were rooted in fantasy. Withers and Mitchell (1995) were concerned that, once again, genuine survivors would not be believed, and I would add to this that there is a danger that the immense difficulties survivors are already faced with when considering disclosure could be compounded.

A clinical and research update on recovered memories of abuse by Brown (1997) attempted to answer a number of pertinent questions. First, there was the issue of whether trauma can be forgotten and later recalled. Here, reference was made with respect to the available empirical data that indi-cated that there were circumstances in which people who had experienced trauma had delayed recall of part or all of the event. This was found to be the case not only for trauma experienced, for example, in combat and road traffic accidents, but more specifically as a result of CSA (Williams, 1994; Elliot and Briere, 1994, 1995; Koss et al, 1994; Scheflin and Brown, 1996). With respect to this particular update, Brown (1997) concluded that the general consensus was that memories of childhood abuse can indeed be lost from and later returned to conscious recollection. The second question that was addressed was about the existence of a false memory syndrome. Here, it was unequivocally stated that such a syndrome did not exist. More importantly, referring to Pope's (1996) literature review on the subject, and also the work of Salter (1995), the point was made that all of the so-called "false memory" cases were so labelled by third parties, usually those accused of abusing the individual who brought the charge. Further, the unreliability of perpetrators' testimony was highlighted in view of the fact that denials occur even when there is indisputable evidence (e.g. DNA samples and videotapes) that sexual abuse has occurred.

The third issue addressed in Brown's review was the argued possibility that false memories of CSA can be easily implanted using psychother-apeutic techniques. The author throws reasonable doubt on the possibility that false memories can be "implanted" and supports her doubt by sug-gesting that the conclusion reached by some that this process is feasible is based on a questionable premise. For example, the work of Loftus (1993), which suggested that false memories can be implanted, was criticised by Pope and Brown (1996) as well as Hyman (1996), for using material that cannot be considered analogous to CSA (i.e. employing the example of two cases of older siblings who managed to convince their younger siblings that they were lost in a shopping mall when they were young). The pertinent point was made by these authors that such examples cannot be considered to be analogous to CSA because they do not contain the burden of having to challenge beliefs about family relationships and are free of social stigma. Brown's (1997) update on recovered memories, however, concluded by highlighting the rapidly changing state of knowledge and science in that area, and alerted clinicians to the need for continuing education, and active consultation towards responsible and effective practice.

The latest report on recovered memories by the American Psychological Association's working group (Alpert et al, 2000) mostly reiterates the 1997 conclusions that most people who have experienced CSA remember all or part of this experience and that it is possible to recollect memories of abuse that have hitherto been forgotten. They do, however, point out that it is possible to construct "pseudo-memories" for events that never occurred—a point that is at odds with Brown's (1997) conclusion on this issue, and one that clearly highlights the changing nature of this topic. Finally, the authors rightly point out that the controversy surrounding the recovered/false memory debate, should not distract attention from the fact that there exists a very real problem in terms of children who are sexually abused, and that there are still substantial gaps in our current knowledge. With respect to implications for therapists, the authors of this recent report offer the following cautionary remarks: although it is necessary that therapists include explicit questions about the history of CSA during intake procedures, when recovered memories are suspected, clients should be informed about treatment alternatives, in terms of benefits, relative risks, and evidence for efficacy; hypnosis is not considered to be an appropriate procedure for exploring or confirming recollections, particularly in view of the fact that this method could jeopardise future legal actions due to its lack of credibility; finally, the point is made that the first goal of treatment, when recollection of trauma occurs, should be to stabilise the situation, and that, in general, recollection of trauma is not necessarily helpful unless it is believed to be necessary for improved functioning and integration of the individual.

MY EXPERIENCE

I hope the reader will appreciate that the background to the false/recovered memory debate presented in the previous section is by no means inclusive of all the information we have to date. This was deliberate on my part because I did not wish to move the focus away from what has been the essential aim of this book: to validate the experience of survivors of CSA and accord them a fair hearing and respect. I would like to make clear, however, that I have presented the above summary in a manner that accords due attention to those issues I consider to be of particular relevance to practitioners. Indeed, it is essentially in my role as practitioner that I shall be discussing the issues raised in the first section in relation to my own clinical work. In this sense, I do not aspire to anything more than to present the picture as I have experienced it and do not wish to undermine the efforts of scientific work in this very complex and recent area of research.

I have always believed unequivocally that the business of psychological practice carries with it great responsibility, and my primary motive has been to be of help to those who seek therapy in order to alleviate their suffering. In this sense, I am not a detective nor a policeman who seeks to extract historical truth out of my clients, be they survivors of sexual abuse or not. At the same time, I would not be an empathic, responsible, and trustworthy therapist if I did not allow my clients to narrate their story in a manner they chose and, therefore, acknowledging their pain assumes superiority over the collation of facts. I would argue that this is not a unique premise—quite the contrary—and I believe that most trained therapists aspire to the same rules. It is true that there are people who set up in practice without appropriate qualifications and this is always of great concern, but for the moment let us remain with those who have earned their practitioner's title.

In the initial stages of the recovered memory debate a great deal of criticism was meted out at certain types of therapy uncovering abuse, and towards therapists (particularly those treating survivors of CSA), which gave the impression that such therapists almost sought out memories of abuse in their clients, whether or not they existed; indeed, some well-known practitioners in this field were actually singled out for criticism (Lindsay and Read, 1994). I share the discomfort experienced by other clinicians as a result of this arguably glib attack, and feel that I, too, am at a loss as to why any therapist would go about instilling further distress, not to mention dependence, in their clients. I, like many clinical psychologists not in private practice, work in an already overstretched service and, in the past decade, have personally assessed in the region of 2,500 patients. At least two-thirds of these patients have received some form of psychological intervention and a significant minority was offered long-term therapy, which, in some instances, lasted for up to three years.

The next important observation refers to the fact that the majority of survivors I have seen had already disclosed their CSA to someone else. Indeed, for a substantial number of survivors, particularly in the "coping very badly" and "coping badly" categories (see Chapter 5), there is usually corroboration of the existence of CSA from previous reports, such as social services, psychiatric notes, perpetrators' conviction, and, of course, current family members and friends. In the relatively few instances where the abuse was disclosed during the course of therapy, this did not occur during an attempt to "uncover memories", but rather, the survivor considered herself to be comfortable enough and trusting of the therapeutic relationship to make the disclosure, having been in full awareness of it from the start. In this sense, I have never experienced a patient undergo a sudden "flash of light" effect in the consulting room, which made them realise that they had been abused. On the other hand, it is not uncommon for survivors to recollect further details of an abusive experience once they have been engaged in therapy. This recollection is certainly not unique to CSA, because other patients are equally able to complete their personal story during the therapeutic process.

A further point that requires highlighting concerns patients' resistance to accepting unequivocally a therapist's suggestions or formulations. In the case of CSA in particular, my experience has been that survivors' striving for control and their understandable mistrust of others does not allow them to be automatically open to suggestions, even if they are made by professionals. Indeed, bearing in mind the difficulties involved in attempting to change people's behaviour, let alone personal beliefs and attitudes, I find it difficult to envisage the extent of power a particular therapist and his/her technique would have in order to instil in someone the belief that they had experienced a substantial trauma, never previously considered by them. That is not to negate the substantial influence that a therapist can have on a patient, particularly when a sound collaborative relationship has been established. Indeed, I personally feel considerably more effective with a survivor when I have managed to engage her and when she trusts me sufficiently to begin discussing issues of a personal and painful nature. In this sense, I prefer to see myself as a helpfully influential guide rather than someone who has power to make my patient change or to render her "suggestible" to my propositions.

Occasionally, a patient might wish to discuss with me the possibility that she may have been sexually abused. I would never advocate embarking on an investigative trail to prove or disprove her suspicion, but will, instead, address the reasons for this request. It is not uncommon, for example, for patients who have had a particularly difficult childhood and who are unable to recall all of the sequence of this childhood to make a reasonable assumption that something sinister may have happened to them. This speculation is fully understandable even though it may be incorrect. There is a natural inclination in all of us to try and make sense of our suffering and, given the huge recent coverage of sexual abuse and its consequences in the media and popular literature, it is easy to appreciate how a person who has suffered as a child might reach the conclusion that they were abused.

The task of a responsible therapist is to engage patients in a collaborative discussion about their suspicion and to identify current areas of difficulty that might require immediate intervention in order, in the first instance, to increase personal efficacy. It is also important that the patient is provided with information about therapeutic techniques and an explanation about their limitations and contra-indications. For example, I was asked on a handful of occasions whether I could use hypnotic regression in order to ascertain whether CSA had taken place. This particular therapeutic technique is not one I have ever contemplated (even before the debate in question), simply because I was never satisfied that it had a sound empirical base, and personally I have never felt comfortable with the notion of assuming a position of doubtful therapeutic "power", since the patient is inevitably a passive collaborator. I have also always assumed that such a situation would clearly be at odds with the importance of helping survivors to become empowered and to be active collaborators who have been duly equipped by the therapist to provide informed consent for their treatment.

The reader will recall that I employed the technique of "guided imagery with rescripting" in two of the case studies. In order to reassure readers who have encountered some criticism of this technique (e.g. Lindsay and Read, 1994), I would like to assert that it has subsequently been acknowledged as a very effective tool (Smucker et al, 1995; Arntz and Weertman, 1999). I have found guided imagery to be particularly effective in two types of situation: when a survivor is prevented from progressing due to persistent post-traumatic effects, such as images, nightmares, and flashbacks; and, secondly, when a particular theme from their childhood—e.g. feeling of abandonment or emotional deprivation—has not been effectively addressed by cognitive techniques. I dispute Lindsay and Read's (1994) contention that the "script" to be addressed is provided by the therapist. Indeed, Young (1994) clearly states that the therapist invites the patient to supply the "script" that most depicts the source of their distress (see, Victoria and Rose, Chapters 9 and 10 respectively). More importantly, guided imagery requires that the patient is a fully active collaborator in a task that does not involve covert or suggestive principles.

In less than a handful of occasions I was involved in cases when a false accusation of sexual abuse was made towards a parent. These were distressing situations for all involved, and they highlight the need for expertise and sensitivity in those who are handling them. These cases, however, were not the result of recovered memories, but of a consciously fabricated lie by the person who made the accusation, usually an adolescent girl. Such cases are very challenging as they generally involve a number of professional agencies due to the acute concern for the safety of the minor and the distress that is being caused to the parents, and of course the latter's possible culpability. In my own experience, these false accusations were eventually retracted, and it transpired that the patients had significant personality problems that were being exacerbated by their perception of neglect and invalidation. While the need for attention in such patients is immense, it is not unusual to discover at some later stage that sexual abuse had occurred at the hands of a non-family member.

It is not difficult to be empathic towards the parents of patients who have been falsely accused. I have, myself, observed their devastation and their attempts at rebuilding their lives following the traumatic experience and public exposure. However, such incidents have been rare when measured against the sheer number of patients I have seen, and I am always struck by the disproportional extent of unacknowledged genuine incidents of CSA, which far exceed the cases where a false accusation has been made.

This discussion raises the issue of legal proceedings when a disclosure of CSA is brought into the public arena. In Chapter 4 I explained that in my own therapeutic involvement with CSA, the frequency of survivors choosing to make an official complaint in adult life was extremely low. Out of 180 women, only thirty-three made such complaints, and only a very small number of these commenced proceedings during the course of therapy. Indeed, most had already provided written statements to the police and it was the distress experienced during this process that led them to seek, or be referred for, help. Interestingly, although the compilation of psychological reports, particularly in the area of compensation for damages, is an integral part of my work, I have never to date been requested to appear as expert witness for any of my clients in relation to allegations of CSA, and to my knowledge no such evidence was sought. This may be partly due to the fact that very few cases actually reached the courts, and also because most court proceedings had already taken place in a different constituency. The important fact remains, however, that as things stand the American Psychiatric Association's working group on recovered memories has recently recommended that it is preferable that therapists do not act as expert witnesses for their clients (see Alpert et al, 2000), given the controversy that surrounds the issue of recovered memories. It is clearly an area where one awaits further empirical opinion.

I wish to conclude this chapter by making two general, but nevertheless, important observations. It is my opinion that there is no magical or sudden process that leads to the realisation that a person has been abused. My extensive experience in this area leads me to speculate that, in general, survivors have differing states of "readiness" that allow them to begin the emotional and cognitive processing of their painful experiences, be they related to sexual abuse or other perceived trauma. This readiness encompasses a host of factors relating to developmental, maturational, psychological, social, and cultural circumstances.

Finally, instead of attacking "quasi therapists" whose training might not be up to scratch, I prefer to propose that the whole field of CSA be accorded the respect it deserves by elevating it to a discreet area of study and training (i.e. in universities and clinical training centres). I have yet to attend a major academic conference symposium solely devoted to the topic of CSA. The latter is at best the poor relation, relegated to an allied topic with greater academic status. How will we continue to increase our understanding of this hugely complex and emotive area unless we accord it serious consideration? I believe there is an urgent need for change.

Chapter 15

An uncertain future: The resilience of paedophilia and the role of society

"Why do people sexually abuse children?" and "Why was my abuse not stopped?" are two poignant questions repeatedly asked by survivors. While we are still some distance away from being able to provide satisfactory answers, in this final chapter I present, in brief, some of the theoretical arguments put forward regarding the psychology of child sex offenders, and also the measures adopted by various caring professions and law enforcement agencies towards child protection.

CHILD SEX OFFENDERS

Writing this section has been extremely difficult. The literature I covered has not by any means succeeded, in my opinion, in providing a wholly satisfactory answer to the survivors' question, "Why do people sexually abuse children"? For a start, a recent article in the *Behavioural Science and the Law* journal (Stone et al, 2000) points out that it is important not to lump all child sex offenders under the umbrella of paedophilia. The writers further argue that distinguishing between paedophilia (sexual attraction to children), sex offences involving children, and the sexual abuse of children, can have far-reaching implications in legal and sentencing terms.

Reading this paper highlighted the first confusion that currently exists, because, particularly in the popular media, the term paedophilia appears to have become the generic term referring to all child sex offences. It is also generally assumed, however, that a person can be a paedophile in fantasy and thought without succumbing to the actual abuse of children. In the psychiatric context, paedophilia is subsumed under the class of sexual disorders termed paraphilias and is defined as, "gross impairment in the capacity for affectionate sexual activity between adult human partners" (Merck Manual, 1992). Further potential confusion, particularly in the eyes of survivors, may arise from the DSM-IV's (American Psychiatric Association, 1994) definition of paraphilias, which also includes paedophilia, as follows: "recurrent, intense sexually arousing fantasies, sexual urges, or behaviours generally involving: (a) non-human objects; (b) the suffering or humiliation of oneself or one's partner; or (c) children or other non-consenting persons, that occur over a period of a least six months". Given this definition, where would an offender who abuses a child on one occasion only, or several occasions during a period of less than six months, fit into this category? Are they actually paedophiles or child sex offenders?

In spite of these complexities, the aim of this chapter is to attempt some explanations with reference only to child sex offenders and in the context of survivors' experience and concerns, and I outline, briefly, the conceptual frameworks I have found to be of particular relevance. In 1984, Finkelhor outlined a set of four preconditions leading to the abuse of children, whereby perpetrators would: (a) have a motivation to abuse a child sexually; (b) need to overcome internal inhibitions against acting on that motivation; (c) need to overcome external constraints to committing the abuse; and (d) need to overcome the child's resistance to being abused. Although these preconditions might explain the path to abuse, they are insufficient in providing an understanding of psychological antecedents to sex offenders' sexual desires. More pertinently, they bring to attention the fact that we have yet to identify the mediating factors between the perpetrators' negotiation of these conditions and their translation to actual acts of sexual abuse.

Marshall et al (2000) have recently extended the critique on the relationship between adult attachments and child molestation, by looking at coping variables in perpetrators of CSA and their childhood parental attachments. In reviewing the previous relevant literature, they summarise the following: sexual offenders are likely to experience insecure and/or dysfunctional adult attachment styles (Ward et al, 1995; Ward et al, 1996; Bumby and Hansen, 1997; Smallbone and Dadds, 1998); chronic inadequacy in intimacy and also loneliness (Marshall, 1993; Seidman et al, 1994; Garlick et al, 1996; Marshall and Hambley, 1996; Bumby and Hansen, 1997); and, as children, sexual offenders are more likely to have experienced CSA, usually at the hands of family members (Hanson and Slater, 1988; Dhawan and Marshall, 1996). In line with the latter, a separate study (Haapasalo et at, 1999) not only highlighted the fact that up to 30 per cent of sex offenders have experienced CSA, but that this figure may be a gross underestimate because only 16 per cent of men viewed their experiences as sexual abuse even when the CSA was previously documented. More importantly, perpetrators' age when their own CSA occurred, as well as the abusive acts they experienced, have been reported to be similar to those of their victims (Groth and Burgess, 1979).

In their current study, Marshall et al (2000), employing the Childhood Attachment Questionnaire on 30 child sex offenders, with 24 non-sexual offenders and 29 non-offenders as controls, suggested that while all subjects reported better relationships with their mothers than with their fathers, poor coping was significantly, but not conclusively, related to insecure maternal attachments. Unfortunately, the writers make no clear distinctions in relation to this variable between the three groups of subjects employed, and also acknowledge the limitations of their study. They, nevertheless, provide useful comments in relation to child molesters and implications for treatment. For example, they suggest that the latter are highly self-preoccupied individuals who attempt to control emotional distress by fantasising and daydreaming. The writers go further to propose that child molesters make use of emotion-focused coping, particularly at times of stress, by adopting a "cognitively deconstructed" state, which ensures that immediate and concrete needs are gratified, irrespective of the inappropriateness of their actions. More crucially, McKibben et al (1994) and also Proulx et al (1996), in seeking to illustrate the links between emotion-focused coping, stressful events, and offensive sexual behaviours, found that sexual offenders' masturbatory practices using deviant fantasy material was enhanced in situations involving emotional and interpersonal conflict.

Marshall et al (2000) conclude their study by suggesting that in an effort to treat child molesters it is important not only to address deficits in behavioural and cognitive skills, but also to train them in replacing emotion-focused responses with more task-focused strategies. Moreover, the writers stress the importance of diminishing reliance on fantasy-led sexual activity that could direct actual sexual offending, and interfering with establishing appropriate intimate adult relationships. Marshall et al's critique may be argued to concur with a more psychoanalytic stance, which views extreme aspects of frustrated and fragile masculinity in which appropriate channels of sexual expression are denied due to the repression of emotions and intimate connections, as seeking the least threatening outlet—i.e. sex with a child (e.g. Frosh, 1993).

Another aspect of child sex offenders that has received a great deal of attention concerns their cognitive distortions. These refer to attitudes and beliefs that child molesters adopt in defence of their behaviour (Salter, 1988; Murphy, 1990; Gudjonsson, 1990; Blumenthal et al, 1999). Indeed, in 1989 Barnard et al proposed that cognitive distortions in this group of offenders resulted in deviant sexual fantasies that had the potential of instigating the seeking out of an appropriate victim and eventual offending. Previously, Abel et al (1984) found the following cognitive distortions among child molesters: because children do not disclose to others that they are having sex with a parent, it means they are enjoying it and want it to continue; having sex with children is a good way of teaching them about sexual matters; because children ask adults about sex it means that they want to have sex with them; and children who do not resist an adult's sexual advances must therefore really want sex.

Unfortunately, there is a lack of empirical work linking the above rationalisations to specific variables relating to individual circumstances, criminal behaviours, personality factors, and psychiatric history of perpetrators of CSA. Defining the cognitive style of such offenders may go some way towards explaining the initiation and perpetuation of their acts, but it does not offer an in-depth understanding of their impulse and lack of control towards their offending.

Further comments and conclusions

This section sought to provide some explanations about the behaviour of child sex offenders. The aim was not to engage in a detailed discussion of this topic, but I considered it important to include this brief section, given the survivors' unanimous bewilderment as to why some people abuse children. Although the definitions, theories, and approaches discussed above offer some understanding, I have found them to have limitations that highlight one's awareness that we are still some distance from an in-depth knowledge about the psychology of child sex offenders. For example, I illustrated the potential confusions arising from the use of the word paedophile. While a great deal of attention has recently been focused on those paedophiles who actually carry out sexual abuse on children, we are not yet clear as to why or how other paedophiles who may have similar desires, fantasies and urges, do not actually go on to abuse. Empirical work in this area has the potential of providing important clues as to the mediating factors that translate fantasy into action.

A further issue requiring attention relates to the gender of child sex abusers. Although women as perpetrators have received some attention in recent years (e.g. Wilkins, 1990; Lawson, 1993; Sinason, 1993; Saradjian, 1997; Lewis and Stanley, 2000), it is important to bear in mind that as far as the available empirical and clinical evidence is concerned, the reporting of CSA at the hands of women is significantly lower than that reported for male perpetrators. My first observation on this is that it may be argued the reason for this disproportional representation is that the notion of CSA at the hands of mothers is so abhorrent that not only does it escapes detection, but even the survivors of such abuse are unable to bring themselves to report it. Secondly, adult male survivors of CSA continue to be clinically under-represented and, therefore, this may prevent a more accurate measurement of gender representation.

These last two observations were included in anticipation of critical comment, and taking into account what we know so far as well as my own clinical experience, I would argue that the sexual abuse of children is largely perpetuated by men. Indeed, in line with the latter, my third observation is the fact that women have not been shown to nurture and/or pursue their fantasies and abuse of children with the same degree of motivation as men. Most notably, the uncovering of paedophile rings, and the exploitation of the current advances in communications technology (e.g. the internet), affording paedophiles better access to each other and to more daring avenues for the exploitation and degradation of children, centres almost exclusively on male offenders. Fourthly, child abductions and sadistic murders for the sexual gratification of offenders is almost exclusively a male dominated domain. There are, of course, the female offenders who became notorious in the last century, but these numbered less than a handful.

Turning to the management of child sex offenders, there is great variability in public opinion regarding what should be done with these offenders, and with the advent of greater openness and media reporting of CSA over the past decade, social attitudes have become bolder but not always, necessarily, well informed. It is not unusual to hear calls for the castration and permanent incarceration of child sex offenders, and we have all witnessed on television the power of mob rule. This state of affairs is unfortunate because it succeeds only in perpetuating the myth that child sex offenders are anonymous monsters who prey on small children. While such monsters obviously exist, it is the sex offender within a "normal" family that continues to escape attention, and society is unwilling to confront the distasteful but very real issue that most CSA occurs in the family home.

Interestingly, the survivors whom I have treated have expressed more considered concerns about what should be done to the perpetrators of their abuse. Two very distinctive wishes have come across in the consulting room: one calls for greater justice in the legal process, as well as better-informed ways of conducting the court process; the other, and equally important, calls for greater availability of rehabilitation programmes for offenders in order to prevent further abuse.

There has been no evidence that a cure for sexually deviant behaviour exists, and the general consensus among professionals working in this area has been that the best one can aim for is a reduction in reoffending (e.g. Foa and Emmelkamp, 1983; Perkins, 1993; Moore et al, 1999). The complexity of a discussion about the political, social, financial, and legal constraints that beset the establishing of rehabilitation programmes, as well as the accessing of them for child sex offenders, is such that it would be beyond the scope of this book. Suffice it to say that the issues discussed in this section have highlighted the need for greater clarity in categorising offenders as well as the continued commitment towards increasing our psychological understanding of perpetrators of child sexual abuse.

SOCIETY AND CHILD PROTECTION

In 1989, following various enquiries into child protection, the new Children's Act sought to reform current practices, and suggested that the interests of the child must have primary importance over that of parents, but awareness (particularly in the UK) of the need for organised, multidisciplinary child protection initiatives targeting the general population of children has only acquired momentum in the past seven years. However, on reviewing recent developments in this area I was struck by the dearth of professional publications and official reports from the UK (e.g. MacLeod, 1997; Sanders, 1999), as opposed to the more active contributions from the US (Burgess and Wurtele, 1998; Wurtele 1999; Mulryan et al, 2000; Waldfogel, 2000), The Netherlands (e.g. Taal and Edelaar, 1997), and Ireland (e.g. MacIntyre and Carr, 1999). Considering that the evidence about the prevalence of CSA began to emerge more than a decade earlier, one cannot but be somewhat aghast at this state of affairs. One usually assumes that relevant agencies (e.g. social services, education, medical and healthcare professionals, and law enforcement agencies) are, in principle, highly motivated towards initiating appropriate measures for the protection of vulnerable children, and that a good level of multidisciplinary collaboration exists. In practice, however, it is difficult to gauge the extent to which such tightly organised multidisciplinary projects exist with regard to children who have not come to the attention of social and healthcare agencies. There is also a lack of knowledge about national variations in terms of adoption of child protection measures, and more pertinently, the degree of efficacy that such measures have achieved.

In defence of the current state of affairs is the fact that (a) the extent and long-term effects of CSA is a continually developing area of knowledge, (b) that social reforms are seldom immediate, and, of course, (c) that financial constraints and lack of resources are always mentioned when these reforms are slow in being implemented. It may also be argued that while child protection has of course existed in one form or another for some while, until recently this has been considered to be, principally, the domain of social services and to some extent charitable organisations (e.g. the 1999 NSPCC "Full Stop" campaign and ChildLine). Multi-agency child protection projects, therefore, which include organisations such as education, nursing, medicine, and family centres, may be viewed as the necessary pilots at this stage. Certainly, I have been unable to find any outcome studies evaluating the long-term success of CSA prevention in a wider context as a result of specific child protection measures.

Some relevant contributions

In a very informative paper, Taal and Edelaar (1997) highlight the fact that, despite the common objective in CSA prevention programmes, there is a lack of consensus about which is the best approach. One such variation relates to the types of population targeted—for example, educators only (i.e. parents, teachers, and day care workers), both children and educators, or children only. The central themes in projects targeting primarily children are learning to identify potential abuse situations, adopting adequate responses, and being encouraged to tell a trusted adult (Daro and McCurdy, 1994; Warden, 1996). Taal and Edelaar (1997) rightly emphasise, however, that the types of abusive encounters usually "played out" in these programmes are a pale reflection of the types of incestuous and long-standing abuse that may be experienced by some children. They also make the very pertinent point that in teaching children self-protective measures, this may inadvertently communicate a burden of responsibility that may lead children to feel guilty and inadequate, particularly if they are in an abusive situation that they are unable to stop.

In Dublin, MacIntyre and Carr (1999) have evaluated the effectiveness of a "stay safe primary prevention programme" for CSA in children aged seven and ten years. Primarily, the authors emphasise the importance of teaching children assertiveness skills because studies of child sex offenders have suggested that they can prevent CSA from occurring (Conte et al, 1989; Elliot et al, 1995). The authors point out the variability in content and effectiveness of "stay safe" programmes and argue that positive results are enhanced when parents are also involved because the principles of remaining safe may be further reinforced. MacIntyre and Carr's (1999) format utilised affective, cognitive, and behavioural dimensions of assertiveness and employed a variety of media for greater impact. Although the results of the study suggest that the children who received the training "did better" than those who did not, this improvement appears to be based, largely, on issues of self-esteem and better knowledge about how to remain "safe". It may be argued, however, that while these improvements are desirable and may help a child in the playground through increased self-confidence, it cannot necessarily be assumed that these children will be able to implement the techniques learned when experiencing coercion of a sexual nature, particularly when this occurs at the hands of a trusted parent, relative, or family friend. While one does not wish to discourage the implementation of educational programmes that enhance awareness of personal safety, body ownership, self-esteem, and assertiveness in children, it is, nevertheless, important to remain vigilant to the fact that the overwhelming majority of CSA is intrafamilial. Unfortunately, the vast majority of education packages I have reviewed appear to place the main focus on extrafamilial, or "stranger" abuse.

The summarised concerns of a recent review of the child protection system in the US (Waldfogel, 2000) can be argued to be relevant to at least the most populated and stretched social service catchment areas in the UK. The paper begins by asserting that the social services system is facing a crisis and that it needs urgent reform. This immediately brings to mind a recent public outcry in the media when an eight-year-old girl from west Africa died in London following years of the most horrific neglect and abuse at the hands of her relatives, despite numerous alarm bells raised by various professionals and despite her being registered with her local social service department.

Waldfogel (2000) proposes five recommendations for reform addressing the following:

1. *Over-inclusion*: i.e. the inappropriate inclusion of low-risk families resulting in fewer resources being available to children who are at serious risk.
2. *Under-inclusion*: this is the situation whereby families whose children are at high risk of abuse are not included either due to lack of reporting, or because potential reporters do not feel that the family will receive appropriate help, or because such families are not considered to have crossed the line into serious neglect and abuse.
3. *Service orientation*: this refers to tensions that arise as a result of implementing child protection strategies that do not take into account the needs of specific families.
4. *Service delivery*: this refers to variations in service delivery across communities and the problem of not only reaching ethnic minorities, but of actually being able to provide effective help due to language barriers and cultural differences.
5. *Capacity*: this refers to the fact that the huge increase in the number of child abuse reports over the past 20 years, and the increase in the seriousness of many cases, far exceed the capacity and resources of the current system.

Discussion and final observations

My aim in this discussion has not been to present an exhaustive critique about the current state of child protection for the prevention of CSA within the wider context of the population of children. I did intend, however, to bring to the reader's attention the fact that this is a continually evolving field of work that urgently requires more empirical and practical study. More specifically, there is a need for better communication and liaison between parents and the relevant institutions involved with children concerning the choice and method of implementing child protection strategies. I also, briefly, pointed out some of the potential benefits as well as pitfalls of education-based programmes aimed at increasing children's confidence, safety awareness, and assertiveness skills. One particular concern I have, for example, is the general emphasis being placed on extrafamilial abuse when all the available evidence points to intrafamilial abuse as occurring more frequently.

In closing this chapter, and indeed this book, I wish to assert that the issue of child protection is one that should concern and involve us all. It is ironic that people will go to any lengths to protect their properties and material goods, as exemplified by media campaigns and neighbourhood watches, while one could not possibly envisage watches being organised in an attempt to protect children, or indeed to report suspected abuse to the appropriate agencies. That is not to say that members of the general public do not, on occasion, raise the alarm, but such instances occur in a haphazard manner and any suggestion that organised neighbourhood watches should exist would be surely met with alarm. Of course I am not advocating that such a system be put in place, simply because it stands a reasonable chance of being abused and exploited by certain people who may have other scores to settle, rather than being solely motivated by altruistic reasons. More importantly, there would be an invasion of people's privacy to an extent that might cause distress far outweighing instances of detection of CSA.

So, how do we in society as a whole ensure that we play our part in ensuring that children are sufficiently protected from an ill that is unlikely to abate and has every chance of achieving greater momentum? I cannot pretend to know the answers. As a trainee clinical psychologist I took the cowardly way out by opting to work with adults, even though my primary interest was in working with children. I very quickly realised during my placements that in trying to help children one had an impossible task, feeling impotent that however hard one tried, the family circumstances ultimately dictated the outcome of any intervention, certainly in the long term. Of course, there were the successful instances when families were insightful and prepared to collaborate, but this is not the case for all children, and particularly not for those who are experiencing the most severe level of intrafamilial neglect and abuse. In the end, I rationalised my decision by telling myself that working with adults placed the burden of responsibility for change in their hands, and that hopefully this might enhance their parental capabilities. Fortunately, I have been able to observe this process in numerous instances during my work over the past decade.

I have come full circle back to families and their responsibilities, and this of course concerns us all, either as parents, carers, or helping professionals. But I believe that there is another significant force at work—the intangible state of general values and beliefs that exist as a function of the prevailing culture. One example is the popular media, which appears to revel in sensationalist articles (see Chapter 2) and is, therefore, not necessarily a good vehicle for informed understanding of CSA. While such articles may have increased awareness about CSA and may have encouraged survivors to come forward, they deter us from addressing the real issues about sexual abuse, such as having to admit that most abuse occurs in the home. In other instances, the media may exploit avenues that communicate mixed messages about where we stand in relation to children's sexuality. I am referring here to a recent publication of a new national magazine for "preteens", specifically aimed at girls, which aroused considerable controversy. For example, some people considered the contents to be exploitative of prepubescent girls due to the sexualised tone of the images portrayed. To make matters worse, the first issue was published almost simultaneously with media articles about the uncovering of a large paedophile ring which was using the internet to circulate obscene images of children as young as three years of age.

Clearly, there are numerous issues to be addressed, and it is not sufficient to be seen to be making the right noises where the protection of children from CSA is concerned. We need to be prepared to address the issue with honesty and courage, even when this tests our resources, both emotional and practical. This is undoubtedly and realistically a massive undertaking involving competing forces on both the micro and macro levels of society, but it is nevertheless one that requires urgent and committed attention. Above all, we need to remain vigilant to the fact that the burden of responsibility towards children's safety must lie primarily with adults.

Epilogue

I have attempted to the best of my knowledge, experience and abilities to bring the topic of the aftermath of CSA and the complexities that surround the issue into the twenty-first century. Even as recently as eight years ago, books on adult survivors of CSA would not have contained the controversial and hotly debated topic of false/recovered memories, the role of the media, the dilemmas involved in reforming child protection services, or the difficulties involved in understanding and rehabilitating child sex offenders. This in itself illustrates the changing state of our knowledge and the need to remain focused on this continually evolving area of work. What I have written today may become old news tomorrow.

If am accused of adopting a slightly crusading, personal, or opinionated tone, then I will gladly and proudly accept the accusation, provided I have succeeded in arousing further interest in this topic, and in creating sufficient impetus in others to produce their own work. If nothing else, I hope I have fulfilled my duty in providing a voice to all of the women I have seen and whose exemplary courage merits attention.

Appendix: Recommended reading for treatment issues raised in Chapters 9, 10, and 11

Alexander, P.C. (1992) "Application of attachment theory to the study of sexual abuse", *Journal of Consulting and Clinical Psychology* 60:185–195.

Arntz, A., and Weeterman, A. (1999) "Treatment of childhood memories: Theory and practice", *Behaviour Research and Therapy* 37:714–740.

Christo, G. (1997) "Child sexual abuse: Psychological consequences", *The Psychologist* 10:205–209.

Fennell, M.J.V. (1997) "Low self-esteem: A cognitive perspective", *Behavioural and Cognitive Psychotherapy* 25:1–25.

Firth, M.T. (1997) "Male partners of female victims of child sexual abuse: Treatment issues and approaches", *Journal of Sexual and Marital Therapy* 12:159–171.

Kennerly, H. (2000) *Overcoming Childhood Trauma: A Self Help Guide Using Cognitive Behavioural Techniques*, London: Robinson.

Lange, A., De Beurs, E., Dolan, C., Lachnit, T., Sjollema, S., and Hanewald, G. (1999) "Long-term effects of childhood sexual abuse: Objective and subjective characteristics of the abuse and psychopathology in later life", *The Journal of Nervous and Mental Disease* 187:150–158.

Linehan, M.M. (1998) "Dialectical behaviour therapy for borderline personality disorder", *Clinician's Research Digest*, 19, American Psychological Association.

Resnick, A.P., and Schnicke, M.K. (1993) *Cognitive Processing Therapy for Rape Victims*, London: Sage Publications.

Smucker, M.R., Dancu, C., Foa, E.B. and Niederee, J.L. (1995) "Imagery rescripting: A new treatment for survivors of childhood sexual abuse suffering from post-traumatic stress", *Journal of Cognitive Psychotherapy: An International Quarterly* 9:3–17.

Teasdale, J. (2000) "Prevention of relapse/recurrence in major depression by mindfulness-based cognitive therapy", *Journal of Consulting and Clinical Psychology* 68:615–623.

Young, J.E. (1999, third edition) *Cognitive Therapy for Personality Disorders: A Schema Focused Approach*, Sarasota, Florida: Professional Resource Press.

Young, J.E., and Klosco, J.S. (1993) *Reinventing Your Life*, London: Penguin.

Zanarini, M.C. (1997) *Role of Sexual Abuse in the Etiology of Borderline Personality Disorder*, Washington, DC: American Psychiatric Press.

Notes

2 Fact and fiction

1 Confidentiality and anonymity of survivors has been preserved by changing the names, location, and any details that could compromise them. An additional safeguard has been to incorporate elements of more than one story into each presentation.

4 The survivors: Summary of descriptive variables

1 When missing values appear in any of the tables in this chapter, this indicates that either the women attended for only one session or that they discontinued treatment during the early part of their therapy and, therefore, no detailed history exists. This is due to the fact that the initial sessions do not include a "formal" interview structure in order to allow the survivor to initiate her own agenda. Consequently, information that relates to sexual abuse in particular may not be revealed until several sessions have taken place. On the other hand, some of the missing data may be due to the fact that the women simply did not have the exact answer, and this is the case, specifically, with the following variables: age abuse started; duration of abuse; and frequency of abuse. It should be noted that, although in the majority of referrals the issue of sexual abuse was stated, not all the women wished to address all the details of this during the initial sessions.
2 When small numbers in any category are presented, a detailed breakdown is deliberately avoided in order to maintain confidentiality.

5 Long-term effects of sexual abuse

1 Self-mutilation refers to repeated impulsive episodes of self-harm, often carried out in a ritualised manner and employing a variety of methods of low lethality. Most common are cutting and self-inflicted cigarette burns, but also self-hitting, hair pulling, interfering with wound healing, and scratching. Most of these acts tend to begin in late adolescence or adulthood (Dudo et al, 1997).

6 Model integration and therapeutic alliance

1 The reader will have noted that I have interchangeably used the terms "relationship" and "alliance". I personally favour the term alliance because, while

the notion of relationship is implied in it, it also conveys a contractual premise whereby the survivor and I are equal partners who are willing to cooperate in the process of therapy.

9 Victoria

1 This formulation takes into account that a risk assessment profile has excluded the presence of clinical depression, suicidal ideation, eating disorder, and obsessive compulsive disorder. There was insufficient criteria for the diagnosis of borderline personality disorder.
2 Guided imagery is an experiential technique that does not involve hypnosis. This technique is most effective when clients are unable to resolve emotional material through discourse alone. It must never be used for the elicitation of sexual abuse or any aspects thereof. The "script" to be used must always be chosen by the survivor. For further guidance on this technique refer to the recommended reading list in the Appendix.

13 The survivors' families and the impact of disclosure

1 I have deliberately omitted a discussion of the cases in which three survivors reported CSA at the hands of their mothers. I did so for confidentiality reasons due to the small number of these events and possible ease of identification. Some information regarding women as active paedophiles is included in Chapter 15.

Bibliography

Abel, G.G., Becker, J.V., and Cunningham-Rathner, J. (1984) "Complication, consent, and cognition in sex between children and adults", *Journal of Law and Psychiatry* 7:89–103.

Abroms, E.M. (1983) "Beyond eclecticism", *American Journal of Psychiatry* 140:740–745.

Alexander, P.C. (1992) "Application of attachment theory to the study of sexual abuse", *Journal of Consulting and Clinical Psychology* 60:185–195.

Alpert, J.L., Brown, L.S., Ceci, S.J., Courtois, C.A., Loftus, E.F., and Ornstein, P.A. (2000) "Final report on the American Psychological Association working group on investigation of memories of childhood abuse", *Psychology, Public Policy, and Law* 4:931–1306.

American Psychiatric Association (1987) *Diagnostic and Statistical Manual of Mental Disorders* (third edition), Washington, DC: American Psychiatric Association.

American Psychiatric Association (1994) *Diagnostic and Statistical Manual of Mental Disorders* (fourth edition), Washington, DC: American Psychiatric Press.

Anderson, J., Martin, J., Mullen, P., Romans, S., and Hervison, G.P. (1993) "Prevalence of childhood sexual abuse experiences in a community sample of women", *Journal of the American Academy of Child and Adolescent Psychiatry* 32:911–919.

Andrews, B., Morton, J., Bekerian, D.A., Brewin, C.R., Davies, G.M., and Mollon, P. (1995) "The recovery of memories in clinical practice: Experiences and beliefs of British psychological society practitioners", *The Psychologist* 8:209–214.

Andrews, B., Valentine, R., and Valentine, J.D. (1995) "Depression and eating disorders following abuse in childhood in two generations of women", *British Journal of Clinical Psychology* 34:37–52.

Armstrong, L. (1978) *Kiss Daddy Goodnight: A Speak-Out on Incest*, New York: Pocket Books.

Arntz, A., and Weertman, A. (1999) "Treatment of childhood memories: Theory and practice", *Behaviour Research and Therapy* 37:715–740.

Bagley, C., and Ramsay, R., (1986) "Sexual abuse in childhood: Psychological outcomes and implications for social work practice", *Journal of Social Work and Human Sexuality* 4:33–36.

Baker, A.W., and Duncan, S.P. (1985) "Child sexual abuse: A study of prevalence in Great Britain", *Child Sexual Abuse and Neglect* 9:457–467.

Baker, C.D. (1992) "Female sexuality and health", in P. Nicolson and J.M. Ussher (Eds.) *The Psychology of Women's Health and Health Care*, London: Macmillan.

→ Baker, C.D. (1993) "A cognitive-behavioural model for the formulation and treatment of sexual dysfunction", in J.M. Ussher and C.D. Baker (Eds.) *Psychological Perspectives on Sexual Problems: New Directions in Theory and Practice*, London: Routledge.

Baker, C.D. (1999) "Female survivors of sexual abuse: A study of their experience, survival, and growth". Paper presented to the *Twenty-ninth Annual Congress of the European Association of Behavioural and Cognitive Therapies*, Dresden.

Baker, C.D. (2000) "The experience of childhood sexual abuse: A psychological perspective of adult female survivors in terms of their personal accounts, therapy, and growth", in J.M. Ussher (Ed.) *Women's Health: Contemporary International Perspectives*, London: BPS Books.

Baker, C.D., and de Silva, P. (1988) "The relationship between male sexual dysfunction and belief in Zilbergeld's myths: An empirical investigation", *Sexual and Marital Therapy* 3:229–238.

Barnard, G.W., Fuller, A.K., Robbins, L., and Shaw, T. (1989) *The Child Molester: An Integrated Approach to Evaluation and Treatment*, New York: Brunner/Mazel.

Beck, A.T. (1963) "Thinking and depression: 1, Idiosyncratic content and cognitive distortions", *Archives of General Psychiatry* 9:324–333.

Beck, A.T. (1964) "Thinking and depression: 2, Theory and therapy", *Archives of General Psychiatry* 10:561–571.

Beck, A.T. (1967) *Depression: Causes and Treatment*, Philadelphia: University of Pennsylvania Press.

Beck, A.T. (1976) *Cognitive Therapy and the Emotional Disorders*, New York: International Universities Press.

Beck, A.T., Rush, A.J., Shaw, B.F., and Emery, G. (1979) *Cognitive Therapy of Depression*, New York: Guilford Press.

Beitchman, J., Zucker, K., Hood, J., DaCosta, G., Akman, D., and Cassavia, E. (1992) "A review of the long-term effects of child sexual abuse", *Child Abuse and Neglect* 16:101–118.

Bifulco, A., and Moran, P. (1998) *Wednesday's Child: Research into Women's Experience of Neglect and Abuse in Childhood, and Adult Depression*, London: Routledge.

Binder, R.L., McNeil, D.E., and Goldstone, R.L. (1996) "Is adaptive coping possible for childhood sexual abuse?", *Psychiatric Services* 47:186–188.

Birns, B., and Meyer S.L. (1993) "Mothers' role in incest: Dysfunctional women or dysfunctional theories", *Journal of Child Sexual Abuse* 2:127–135.

Blacke-White, J., and Kline, C.M. (1985) "Treating the dissociative process in adult victims of childhood incest", *Social Casework: The Journal of Contemporary Social Work* 9:394–402.

Blumenthal, S., Gudjonsson, G., and Burns, J. (1999) "Cognitive distortions and blame attribution in sex offenders against adults and children", *Child Abuse and Neglect* 23:129–143.

Bowlby, J. (1973) *Separation: Anxiety and Anger* (Vol. II of *Attachment and Loss*), New York: Basic Books.

Bowlby, J. (1980) *Attachment and Loss*, Vol. III: *Loss, Sadness and Depression*, London: Hogarth Press.

Bowlby, J. (1988) *A Secure Base: Clinical Applications of Attachment Theory*, London: Routledge.

Briggs, L., and Joyce, P. (1997) "What determines post-traumatic stress disorder symptomatology for survivors of childhood sexual abuse?", *Child Abuse and Neglect* 21:575–582.

Brodsky, B.S., Cloitre, M., and Dulit, R.A. (1995) "Relationship of dissociation to self-mutilation and childhood abuse in borderline personality disorder", *American Journal of Psychiatry* 152:1788–1792.

Brown, L.S. (1997) "Recovered memories of abuse: Research and clinical update", *Clinician's Research Digest* 17, American Psychological Association.

Bryer, J.B., Nelson, B.A., Miller, J.B., and Krol, P.A. (1987) "Childhood sexual and physical abuse as factors in adult psychiatric illness", *American Journal of Psychiatry* 144:1426–1430.

Bullough, V.L. (1990) "History in adult human sexual behaviour with children and adolescents in Western societies", in J.R. Feierman (Ed.) *Paedophilia: Biosocial Dimensions*, New York: Springer-Verlag.

Bumby, K.M., and Hansen, D.J. (1997) "Intimacy deficits, fear of intimacy, and loneliness among sexual offenders", *Criminal Justice and Behaviour* 24:315–331.

Burgess, E.S., and Wurtele, S.K. (1998) "Enhancing parent child communication about sexual abuse: A pilot study", *Child Abuse and Neglect* 22:1167 1175.

Cahil, C., Llewelyn, S.P., and Pearson, C. (1991) "Long-term effects of sexual abuse which occurred in childhood: A review", *British Journal of Clinical Psychology* 30:117–130.

ChildLine (2000) "The first twelve years", *Archives of Disease in Childhood* 83:283–285.

Chu, J.A., and Dill, D.L. (1990) "Dissociative symptoms in relation to childhood physical and sexual abuse", *American Journal of Psychiatry* 147:887–892.

Clinician's Research Digest, 19, American Psychological Association.

Coccaro, E.F., Siever, L.J., Klar, H.M., Maurer, G., Cochrane, K., Cooper, T.B., Mohs, R.C., and Davis, K.L. (1989) "Serotonergic studies in patients with affective and personality disorders", *Archives of General Psychiatry* 46:587–599.

Coffey, P., Leitenberg, H., Henning, K., Turner, T., and Bennet, R. (1996) "Mediators of the long-term impact of child sexual abuse: Perceived stigma, betrayal, powerlessness, and self-blame", *Child Abuse and Neglect* 20:447–455.

Colapino, J. (1984) "On model integration and model integrity", *Journal of Strategic and Systemic Therapies* 4:38–42.

Cole, P.M., and Putnam, F.W. (1992) "Effect of incest on self and social functioning: A developmental psychological perspective", *Journal of Consulting and Clinical Psychology* 60:174–184.

Conte, J., Wolfe, S., and Smith T. (1989) "What sexual offenders tell us about prevention strategies", *Child Abuse and Neglect* 13:293–301.

Courtois, C.A. (1988) *Healing the Incest Wound: Adult Survivors in Therapy*, New York: Norton.

Coverdale, J.H., and Turbott, S.H. (2000) "Sexual and physical abuse of chronically ill psychiatric outpatients compared with a matched sample of medical outpatients", *Journal of Nervous and Mental Disease* 188:440–445.

Crawford, S.L. (1999) "Intrafamilial sexual abuse: What we think we know about mothers, and implications for intervention", *Journal of Child Sexual Abuse* 7:55–72.

Dadds, M., Smith, M., Webber, Y., and Robinson, A. (1991) "An exploration of family and individual profiles following father–daughter incest", *Child Abuse and Neglect* 15:575–586.

Daro, D., and McCurdy, K. (1994) "Preventing child abuse and neglect: Programmatic interventions", *Child Welfare* 73:405–430.

Davies, M.G. (1995) "Parental distress and ability to cope following disclosure of extrafamilial sexual abuse", *Child Abuse and Neglect* 19:399–408.

Davis, L. (1991) *Allies in Healing*, New York: Harper Collins.

Department of Health and Social Security (1988) *Cleveland Inquiry*, HMSO: London.

Department of Health (1993) *Children and Young people in Child Protection Registers in England for the Year Ended 31.3.92*, HMSO: London, p. 10.

Dhawan, S., and Marshall, W.L. (1996) "Sexual abuse histories of sexual offenders", *Sexual Abuse: A Journal of Research and Treatment* 8:7–15.

Dickinson, L.M., DeGruy III, F.V., Dickinson, W.P., and Candib, L.M. (1998) "Complex post-traumatic stress disorder: Evidence from the primary care setting", *General Hospital Psychiatry* 20:214–224.

DiLillo, D., and Long P.J. (1999) "Perceptions of couple functioning among female survivors of child sexual abuse", *Journal of Child Sexual Abuse* 7:59–77.

Dudo, E.D., Zanarini, M.C., Lewis, R.E., and Williams, A.A. (1997) "Relationship between lifetime self-destructiveness and pathological childhood experiences", in M.C. Zanarini (Ed.) *Role of Sexual Abuse in the Aetiology of Borderline Personality Disorder*, Washington, DC: American Psychiatric Press.

Dyson, F. (1995) "The scientist as rebel", *New York Review of Books*, 25 May:31.

Edgarth, K., and Ormstad, K. (2000) "Prevalence and characteristics of sexual abuse in a national sample of Swedish 17-year-old boys and girls", *Acta Paediatrica* 89:310–319.

Edwards, J.J., and Alexander, P.C. (1992) "The contribution of family background to the long-term adjustment of women sexually abused as children", *Journal of Interpersonal Violence* 7:306–320.

Edwards, S., and Lohman, J. (1994) "The impact of 'moral panic' on professional behaviour in cases on child sexual abuse: An international perspective", *Journal of Child Sexual Abuse* 3:103–126.

Elliott, D.M., and Briere, J.N. (1994) "Trauma and dissociated memory: Prevalence across events", in L. Berliner (Chair) *Delayed Trauma Memories: Victim Experiences and Clinical Practice*. Symposium presented at the Tenth Annual Meeting, International Society for Traumatic Stress Studies, Chicago, IL.

Elliott, D.M., and Briere, J.N. (1995) "Post-traumatic stress associated with delayed recall of sexual abuse: A general populations study", *Journal of Traumatic Stress* 8:629–647.

Elliott, M., Browne, K., and Kilcoyne, J. (1995) "Child sexual abuse prevention: What offenders tell us", *Child Abuse and Neglect* 19:579–594.

Elvik, S. (1994) "The effect of the media on child sexual abuse: Commentary", *Journal of Child Sexual Abuse* 3:133–135.

Engle, B. (1991) *Partners in Recovery: How Mates, Lovers, and other Prosurvivors Can Learn to Support and Cope with Adult Survivors of Childhood Sexual Abuse*, Los Angeles: Lowell House.

Everill, J., and Waller, G. (1995) "Disclosure of sexual abuse and psychological adjustment in female undergraduates", *Child Abuse and Neglect* 19:93–100.

Eysenck, H.J. (Ed.) (1960) *Behaviour Therapy and Neuroses*, New York: Pergamon Press.

Fallon, P., and Coffman, S. (1991) "Cognitive behavioural treatment of survivors of victimisation", *Psychotherapy in Private Practice* 9:53–64.

Faust, J., Runyon, M.K., and Kenny, M.C. (1995) "Family variables associated with the onset and impact of intrafamilial childhood sexual abuse", *Clinical Psychological Review* 15:443–456.

Feltham, C. (Ed.) (1999) *Understanding the Counselling Relationship*, London: Sage.

Fennell, M.J.V. (1997) "Low self-esteem: A cognitive perspective", *Behavioural and Cognitive Psychotherapy* 25:1–25.

Ferguson, A.G. (1997) "How good is the evidence relating to the frequency of childhood sexual abuse and the impact such abuse has on the lives of adult survivors?", *Public Health* 111, 6:387–391.

Finkelhor, D. (1979) *Sexually Victimised Children*, New York: Free Press.

Finkelhor, D. (1980) "Risk factors in the sexual victimisation of children", *Child Abuse and Neglect* 4:265–273.

Finkelhor, D. (1984) *Child Sexual Abuse: New Theory and Research*, New York: Free Press.

Finkelhor, D. (1988) "The trauma of child sexual abuse: Two models", in G. Wyatt and G. Powell (Eds.) *Lasting Effects of Child Sexual Abuse*, London: Sage.

Finkelhor, D. (1990) "Early and long-term effects of child sexual abuse: An update", *Professional Psychology: Research and Practice* 21:325–350.

Finkelhor, D. (1991) "The scope of the problem", in K. Murray and D. Gough (Eds.) *Intervening in Child Sexual Abuse*, Glasgow: Scottish Academic Press.

Finkelhor, D. (1994a) "The international epidemiology of child sexual abuse", *Child Abuse and Neglect* 18:409–417.

Finkelhor, D. (1994b) "Current information on the scope and nature of childhood sexual abuse", *Future of Children* 4:31–53.

Finkelhor, D., and Browne, A. (1985) "The traumatic impact of child sexual abuse: A conceptualisation", *American Journal of Orthopsychiatry* 66:530–541.

Finkelhor, D., and Browne, A. (1986) "Initial and long-term effects: A conceptual framework", in D. Finkelhor (Ed.) *A Sourcebook on Child Sexual Abuse*, Beverly Hills: Sage.

Finkelhor, D., and Dziuba-Leatherman, J. (1994) "Children as victims of violence: A national study", *Pediatrics* 94:413–420.

Finkelhor, D., Hotaling, G.T., Lewis I.A., and Smith, C. (1989) "Sexual abuse and its relationship to later sexual satisfaction, marital status, religion, and attitudes", *Journal of Interpersonal Violence* 4:379–399.

Firth, M.T. (1997) "Male partners of female victims of child sexual abuse: Treatment issues and approaches", *Journal of Sexual and Marital Therapy* 12:159–171.

Fleming, J. (1998) "Childhood sexual abuse: An update", *Current Opinion in Obstetrics and Gynaecology* 10:383–386.

Fleming, J., Sibthorpe, P., and Bammer, G. (1999) "The long-term impact of childhood sexual abuse in Australian women", *Child Abuse and Neglect* 23:145–159.

Foa, E.B., and Emmelkamp, P.M.G. (1983) *Failures in Behaviour Therapy*, New York: Wiley.

Freud, S. (1920) *Beyond the Pleasure Principle: The Standard Edition of the Complete Psychological Works of Sigmund Freud*, New York: Basic Books, Inc.

Frosh, S. (1993) "The seeds of masculine sexuality", in J.M. Ussher and C.D. Baker (Eds.) *Psychological Perspectives on Sexual Problems: New Directions in Theory and Practice*, London: Routledge.

Garlick, Y., Marshall, W.L., and Thornton, D. (1996) "Intimacy deficits and attribution of blame among sex offenders", *Legal and Criminological Psychology* 1:251–258.

Gil, E. (1992) *Outgrowing the Pain Together: A Book for Spouses and Partners of Adults Abused as Children*, New York: Bentam Books.

Glaser, D., and Frosh, S. (1993) *Child Sexual Abuse*, London: The Macmillan Press Ltd.

Gold, E.R. (1986) "Long-term effects of sexual victimisation in childhood: An attributional approach", *Journal of Consulting and Clinical Psychology* 54:471–475.

Goodwin, J. (1990) "Applying to adult incest victims what we have learned from victimised children", in R.P. Kluft (Ed.) *Incest Related Syndromes of Adult Psychopathology*, Washington, DC: American Psychiatric Press.

Goodwin, J. (1997) "Child abuse: Controversy, sequelae, treatment", *Current Opinion in Psychiatry* 10:432–435.

Gorey, K.M., and Leslie, D.R. (1997) "The prevalence of child abuse: Integrative review adjustment for potential response and measurement biases", *Child Abuse and Neglect* 21:391–398.

Government of the State of New South Wales (1997: PA104) *Final report Vol. VI: The Paedophile Enquiry*, Sydney: Royal Commission into the New South Wales Police Service.

Grogan, S. (2000) "Body image", in J.M. Ussher (Ed.) *Women's Health: Contemporary International Perspectives*, Leicester, UK: BPS Books.

Groth, N.A., and Burgess, A. (1979) "Sexual trauma in the life histories of rapists and child molesters", *Victimology: An International Journal* 4:10–16.

Gudjonsson, G.H. (1990) "Cognitive distortions and blame attribution among paedophiles", *Sexual and Marital Therapy* 5:183–185.

Haapasalo, J., Puupponen, M., and Crittenden, P.M. (1999) "Victim to victimiser: The psychology of isomorphism in a case of recidivist paedophile in Finland", *Journal of Child Sexual Abuse* 7:97–115.

Hall, R. (1985) *Ask Any Woman: An Inquiry into Rape and Sexual Assault*, Bristol: Falling Wall Press.

Hanson, R.K., and Slater, S. (1988) "Sexual victimisation in the history of sexual abusers: A review", *Annals of Sex Research* 1:485–499.

Hart, L.E., Mader, L., Griffith, K., and de Mendonca, M. (1989) "Effects of sexual and physical abuse: A comparison of adolescent inpatients", *Child Psychiatry and Human Development* 21:49–57.

Hartman, C.R., and Burgess, A.W. (1993) "Information-processing of trauma", *Child Abuse and Neglect* 17:47–58.

Herman, J. (1992) *Trauma and Recovery*, New York: Basic Books.

Herman, J.L. (1981) *Father–Daughter Incest*, Cambridge: Harvard University Press.

Herman, J.L. (1986) "Histories of violence in an outpatient population: An exploratory study", *American Journal of Orthopsychiatry* 56:137–141.

Herman, J.L., Perry, J.C., and van der Kolk, B.A. (1989) "Childhood trauma in borderline personality disorder", *American Journal of Psychiatry* 146:490–495.

HMSO 1988 (Department of Health and Social Security) *Cleveland Inquiry*: London.

HMSO 1993 (Department of Health and Social Security) *Children and Young People in Child Protection Registers in England for the Year Ended 31.3.92*, HMSO: London.

Hyman, I.E. (1996) "False childhood memories: Research, theory, and applications". Plenary address to *Trauma and Memory: An International Research Conference*, Family Research Laboratory, Durham, NC.

Jehu, D. (1988) *Beyond Sexual Abuse: Therapy with Women who were Childhood Victims*, Chichester: Wiley.

Jehu, D. (1991) "Post-traumatic stress reactions among adults molested as children", *Sexual and Marital Therapy* 6:227–243.

Jehu, D., Klassen, C., and Gazan, M. (1985/6) "Cognitive restructuring of distorted beliefs associated with childhood sexual abuse", *Journal of Social Work and Human Sexuality* 4:49–69.

Kabat-Zinn, J. (1990) *Full Catastrophe Living*, New York: Delta.

Kennerley, H. (2000) *Overcoming Childhood Trauma: A Self Help Guide Using Cognitive Behavioural Techniques*, London: Robinson.

Kent, A., Waller, G., and Dagnan, D. (1999) "A greater role of emotional than physical or sexual abuse in predicting disordered eating attitudes: The role of meditating variables", *International Journal of Eating Disorders* 25:159–167.

Kirby, J.S., Chu, J.A., and Dill, D.L. (1993) "Correlates of dissociative symptomatology in patients with physical and sexual abuse histories", *Comprehensive Psychiatry* 34:258–263.

Kirschner, S., Kirschner, D.A., and Rappaport, R.L. (1993) *Working with Adult Incest Survivors: The Healing Journey*, New York: Brunner/Mazel.

Koss, M.P., Goodman, L.A., Browne A., Fitzgerald, L.F., Keita, G.W., and Russo, N.F. (1994) *No Safe Haven*, Washington, DC: American Psychiatric Association.

Kristberg, W. (1990) *Healing Together*, Deerfield Beach, FL: Health Communications.

Kubler-Ross, E. (1989) *On Death and Dying*, London: Routledge.

La Barbera, J.D., Martin, J.E., and Dozier, J.E. (1980) "Child psychiatrists' view of father–daughter incest", *Child Abuse and Neglect* 4:147–151.

Landecker, H. (1992) "The role of childhood sexual trauma in the aetiology of borderline personality disorder: Consideration for diagnosis and treatment", *Psychotherapy* 29:234–242.

Lange, A., De Beurs, E., Dolan, C., Lachnit, T., Sjollema, S., and Hanewald, G. (1999) "Long-term effects of childhood sexual abuse: Objective and subjective characteristics of the abuse and psychopathology in later life", *The Journal of Nervous and Mental Disease* 187:150–158.

Lawson, C. (1993) "Mother-on sexual abuse: rare or underrreported? A critique of the research", *Child Abuse and Neglect* 17:261–269.

Levang, C.A. (1989) "Interactional communication patterns in father/daughter incest families", *Journal of Psychology and Human Sexuality* 1:53–68.

Leventhal, J.M. (1998) "Epidemiology of sexual abuse of children: Old problems, new directions", *Child Abuse and Neglect* 22:481–491.

Leventhal, J.M. (2000) "Sexual abuse of children: Continuing challenges of the new millennium", *Acta Paediatrica* 89:268–271.

Levey, B. (1999) "The media", *Child Abuse and Neglect* 23:995–1001.

Lewis, C.F., and Stanley, C.R. (2000) "Women accused of sexual offences", *Behavioural Sciences and the Law* 18:73–81.

Lewis, I.A. (1985) (*Los Angeles Times* Poll no. 98). Unpublished raw data.

Lindberg, F., and Distad, L. (1985) "Post-traumatic stress disorders in women who experienced childhood incest", *Child Abuse and Neglect* 9:329–334.

Lindsay, D.S., and Read, J.D. (1994) "Psychotherapy and memories of childhood sexual abuse: Cognitive perspective", *Applied Cognitive Psychology* 8:281–338.

Linehan, M.M. (1993) *Cognitive-Behavioural Treatment for Borderline Personality Disorder*, New York: Guilford.

Linehan, M.M. (1998) "Dialectical behaviour therapy for borderline personality disorder", *Clinicians Research Digest*, 19, American Psychological Association.

Links, P.S., Steiner, M., Offord, D.R., and Eppel, A. (1988) "Characteristics of borderline disorder: A Canadian study", *Canadian Journal of Psychiatry* 33:336–340.

Lipovsky, J., Saunders, B., and Hanson, R. (1992) "Parent–child relationships of victims and siblings in incest families", *Journal of Child Sexual Abuse* 1:35–49.

Loftus, E.F. (1993) "The reality of repressed memories", *American Psychologist* 48:518–537.

Luborsky, L., Singer, B., and Luborsky, L. (1975) "Comparative studies of psychotherapies: Is it true that 'everyone has won and all must have prizes'", *Archives of General Psychiatry* 32:995–1008.

Lundberg-Love, P.K. (1990) "Adult survivors of incest", in R.T. Ammerman and M. Hersen (Eds.) *Treatment of Family Violence: A Sourcebook*, New York: Wiley.

MacIntyre, D., and Carr, A. (1999) "Evaluation of the effectiveness of the stay safe primary prevention programme for child sexual abuse", *Child Abuse and Neglect* 23:1307–1325.

MacLeod, M. (1997) *Child Protection: Everybody's Business*, London: Reed Business Information/ChildLine.

Macmillan, H.L., Fleming, J.E., Troome, N., Boyle, M.H., Wong, M., Racine, Y.A., Beardslee, W.R., and Offord, D.R. (1997) "Prevalence of child physical and sexual abuse in the community: Results from the Ontario Health Supplement", *Journal of the American Medical Association* 278:131–135.

Malz, W. (1988) "Identifying and treating the sexual repercussions of incest: A couples therapy approach", *Journal of Sex and Marital Therapy* 14:142–170.

Markowitz, P. (1993) "Longitudinal efficacy of SSRI in borderlines". Paper presented at the *Third International Congress on the Disorders of Personality*, Cambridge, MA.

Marks, I. (1986) *Behavioural Psychotherapy*, Bristol: Wright.

Marshall, W.L. (1993) "The role of attachment, intimacy, and loneliness in the etiology and maintenance of sexual offending", *Sexual and Marital Therapy* 8:109–121.

Marshall, W.L., and Hambley, L.S. (1996) "Intimacy and loneliness and their relationship to rape myth acceptance and hostility toward women among rapists", *Journal of Interpersonal Violence* 11:586–592.

Marshall, W.L., Serran, G.A., and Cortoni, F.A. (2000) "Childhood attachments, sexual abuse and their relationship to adult coping in child molesters", *Sexual Abuse: A Journal of Research and Treatment* 12:17–26.

Maslow, A. (1957) *Motivation and Personality*, New York: Harper & Row.

Masson, J.M. (1989) *Against Therapy*, London: Harper Collins.

McConaghy, N. (1998) "Paedophilia: A review of the evidence", *Australian and New Zealand Journal of Psychiatry* 32:252–265.

McGinn, L.K., and Young, J.E. (1996) "Schema-focused therapy", in P.M. Salkovskis (Ed.) *Frontiers of Cognitive Therapy*, New York: Guilford.

McKibben, A., Proulx, J., and Lusignan, R. (1994) "Relationship between conflict, affect and deviant sexual behaviours in rapists and paedophiles", *Behaviour Research and Therapy* 32:571–575.

McLeer, S., Deblinger, E., Atkins, M., Foa, E., and Ralphe, D. (1988) "Post-traumatic disorder in sexually abused children", *Journal of the American Academy of Child and Adolescent Psychiatry* 27:651–654.

Mearns, D., and Thorne, B. (1988) *Person-Centred Counselling in Action*, London: Sage.

Melchert, T.P. (2000) "Maternal acceptance buffers effects of childhood trauma", *Professional Psychology: Research and Practice* 31:64–69.

Mennen, F.E., and Meadow, D. (1994) "A preliminary study of the factors related to trauma in childhood sexual abuse", *Journal of Family Violence* 9:125–142.

"Merck Manual" (1992, 16th edition) *Merck Manual of Diagnosis and Therapy* 1570.

Metcalfe, M. (1994) "Childhood sexual experiences in psychiatric and general practice attenders: The Leicester studies", paper presented at the September *National Conference on Mental Health Aspects of Adult Survivors of Sexual Abuse*.

Miller, B.A., Downs, W.R., and Testa, M. (1993) "Interrelationships between victimisation experiences and women's alcohol use", *Journal of Studies on Alcohol* 11:109–117.

Moore, D.L., Bergman, B.A., and Knox, P.L. (1999) "Predictors of sex offender treatment completion", *Journal of Child Sexual Abuse* 7:73–88.

Morrow, K.B., and Sorrell, G.T. (1989) "Factors affecting self-esteem, depression, and negative behaviours in sexually abused female adolescents", *Journal of Marriage and the Family* 51:677–686.

Mrazek, P., Lynch, M., and Bentovim, A. (1983) "Sexual abuse of children in the United Kingdom", *Child Abuse and Neglect* 7:147–153.

Mullen, P.E., Martin, J.L., Anderson, J.C., Romans, S.E., and Herbison, G.P. (1993) "Childhood sexual abuse and mental health in adult life", *British Journal of Psychiatry* 163:721–732.

Mullen, P.E., Martin, J.L., Anderson, J.C., Romans, S.E., and Herbison, G.P.

(1994) "The effect of child abuse on social, interpersonal, and sexual function in adult life", *British Journal of Psychiatry* 165:35–47.

Mullen, P.E., Romans-Clarkson, S.E., Walton, V.A., and Herbison, G.P. (1988) "The impact of sexual and physical abuse on women's mental health", *The Lancet* 4:841–845.

Mulryan, K., Cathers, P., and Fagin, A. (2000) "Combating abuse, part II: Protecting the child", *Nursing* 30:39–43.

Murphy, W.D. (1990) "Assessment and modification of cognitive distortions in sex offenders", in E.L. Marshall, D.R. Laws, and H.E. Barbaree (Eds.) *Handbook of Sexual Assault: Issues, Theories, and Treatment of the Offender*, New York: Plenum Press.

Nagel, D.E., Putnam, F.W., and Noll, J.G. (1997) "Disclosure patterns of sexual abuse and psychological functioning at a one-year follow-up", *Child Abuse and Neglect* 21:137–147.

Nash, M.R., Hulsey, T.L., Sexton, M.C., Harralson, T.L., and Lambert, W. (1993) "Long-term sequelae of childhood sexual abuse: Perceived family environment, psychopathology, and dissociation", *Journal of Consulting and Clinical Psychology* 61:276–283.

NSPCC (1990) *Research Briefing* 11, London: NSPCC Publications.

NSPCC (2000) *Child Maltreatment in the United Kingdom: A Study of Prevalence of Child Abuse and Neglect*, London: NSPCC Publications.

Ogata, S.N., Silk, K.R., Goodrich, S., Lohr, N.E., Westen, D., and Hill, E.M. (1990) "Childhood sexual and physical abuse in adult patients with borderline personality disorder", *American Journal of Psychiatry* 147:1008–1013.

Oppenheimer, R., Howells, K., Palmer, R.L., and Chaloner, D.A. (1985) "Adverse sexual experience in childhood and clinical eating disorders: A preliminary description", *Journal of Psychiatric Research* 19:357–361.

Pavlov, I.P. (1927) *Conditioned Reflexes*, Oxford: Oxford University Press.

Pedesky, C.A. (1994) "Schema change processes in cognitive therapy", *Clinical Psychology and Psychotherapy* 1:267–278.

Pelletier, G., and Handy, L.C. (1986) "Family dysfunction and the psychological impact of child sexual abuse", *Canadian Journal of Psychiatry* 31:407–412.

Perkins, D. (1993) "Psychological perspectives on working with sex offenders", in J.M. Ussher and C.D. Baker (Eds.) *Psychological Perspectives on Sexual Problems: New Directions in Theory and Practice*, London: Routledge.

Polusny, M.A., and Follette, V.M. (1995) "Long-term correlates of child sexual abuse: Theory and review of the empirical literature", *Applied and Preventive Psychology* 4:143–166.

Pope, K.S. (1996) "Memory, abuse, and science: Questioning claims about the false memory syndrome epidemic", *American Psychologist* 51:957–974.

Pope, K.S., and Brown L.S. (1996) *Recovered Memories of Abuse: Assessment, Therapy, Forensics*, Washington, DC: American Psychological Association.

Pribor, E.F., and Dinwiddie, S.H. (1992) "Psychiatric correlates of incest in childhood", *American Journal of Psychiatry* 149:455–463.

Proulx, J., McKibben, A., and Lusignan, R. (1996) "Relationships between affective components and sexual behaviours in sexual aggressors", *Sexual Abuse: A Journal of Research and Treatment*, 8:279–289.

Rappaport, R.L. (1991) "When eclecticism is the integration of therapist postures, not theories", *Journal of Integrative and Eclectic Psychotherapy* 10:164–172.

Resick, A.P., and Schnicke, M.K. (1992) "Cognitive processing therapy for sexual assault victims", *Journal of Consulting and Clinical Psychology* 60: 748-756.

Resick, A.P., and Schnicke, M.K. (1993) *Cognitive Processing Therapy for Rape Victims*, London: Sage Publications.

Resnick, H., Kilpatrick, D., Danshy, B., Saunders, B., and Best, C. (1993) "Prevalence of civilian trauma and post-traumatic stress disorder in a representative national sample of women", *Journal of Consulting and Clinical Psychology* 61:984–991.

Rogers, C.R. (1951) *Client-Centred Therapy*, Boston: Houghton Mifflin.

Rogers, C.R. (1957) "The necessary and sufficient conditions of therapeutic personality change", *Journal of Counselling Psychology* 21:95–103.

Rogers, C.R. (1959) "A theory of therapy, personality and interpersonal relationships as developed in the client-centred framework", in S. Koch (Ed.) *Psychology: A Study of Science, Vol III: Formulations of the Person and the Social Context*, New York: McGraw-Hill.

Rogers, C.R. (1980) *A Way Of Being*, Boston: Houghton Mifflin.

Rogers, C.R., and Stevens, B. (1973) *Person to Person: The Problem of Being Human*, London: Souvenir Press Ltd.

Romans, S.E., Martin, J.L., and Mullen, P.E. (1996) "Women's self-esteem: A community study for women who report and do not report childhood sexual abuse", *British Journal of Psychiatry*, 169:696–704.

Root, M.P.P., and Fallon, P. (1988) "The incidence of victimisation experiences in a bulimia sample", *Journal of Interpersonal Violence* 3:161 173.

Roth, N. (1993) *Integrating the Shattered Self*, New Jersey: Jason Aronson Inc.

Russell, D.E.H. (1983) "The incidence and prevalence of intrafamilial and extrafamilial sexual abuse of female children", *Child Abuse and Neglect* 7:133–146.

Safran, J.D. (1990) "Towards a refinement of cognitive therapy in the light of interpersonal theory", Parts 1 and 2, *Clinical Psychology Review* 10:87–121.

Safran, J.D. (1996) "Emotion in cognitive behavioural theory and treatment", in P.M. Salkovskis (Ed.) *Trends in Cognitive and Behavioural Therapies*, New York: John Wiley and Sons.

Safran, J.D., Greenberg, L.S., and Rice, L.N. (1988) "Integrating psychotherapy research and practice: Modelling the change process", *Psychotherapy* 25:1–17.

Safran, J.D., and Segal, Z.V. (1990) *Interpersonal Process in Cognitive Therapy*, New York: Basic Books.

Salter, A. (1995) *Transforming Trauma: A Guide to Understanding and Treating Adult Survivors of Child Sexual Abuse*, Thousand Oaks, CA: Sage.

Salter, A.C. (1988) *Treating Child Sex Offenders and Victims: A Practical Guide*, London: Sage Publications.

Salzman, J.P., Salzman, C., Wolfson, A.N., Albanese, M., Looper, J., Ostacher, M., Schwartz, J., Chinman, G., Land, W., and Miyawaki, E. (1993) "Association between borderline personality structure and history of childhood abuse in adult volunteers", *Comprehensive Psychiatry* 34:254–257.

Sanders, D., and Wills, F. (1999) "The therapeutic relationship in cognitive therapy", in C. Feltham (Ed.) *Understanding the Counselling Relationship*, London: Sage.

Sanders, R. (1999) "Child abuse fatalities and cases of extreme concern: Lessons from reviews", *Child Abuse and Neglect* 23:257–268.

Sanderson, C. (1990) *Adul: Survivors of Sexual Abuse*, London: Jessica Kingsley.

Saradjian, J. (1997) *Women Who Sexually Abuse Children: From Research to Clinical Practice*, Chichester: John Wiley & Sons.

Scheflin, A., and Brown, D. (1996) "Repressed memory or dissociative amnesia: What science says", *Journal of Psychiatry and Law* 24:143–188.

Seidman, B.T., Marshall, W.L., Hudson, S.M., and Robertson, P.J. (1994) "An examination of intimacy and loneliness in sex offenders", *Journal of Interpersonal Violence* 9:518–534.

Shearer, S.L., Peters, C.P., Quaytman, M.S., and Ogden, R.L. (1993) "Frequency and correlates of childhood sexual and physical abuse histories in adult female borderline in-patients", *American Journal of Psychiatry* 147:214–216.

Silk, K.R., Nigg, J.T., Westen, D., and Lohr, N.E. (1997) "Severity of childhood sexual abuse, borderline symptoms, and familial environment", in M.C. Zanarini (Ed.) *Role of Sexual Abuse in the Etiology of Borderline Personality Disorder*, Washington, DC: American Psychiatric Press.

Sinason, V. (1993) Talk given at *ChildLine* conference on "Women who sexually abuse children", London.

Skinner, B.F. (1938) *The Behaviour of Organisms: An Experimental Analysis*, New York: Appleton-Century-Croft.

Smallbone, S.W., and Dadds, M.R. (1998) "Childhood attachment and adult attachment in incarcerated adult male sex offenders", *Journal of Interpersonal Violence* 13:555–573.

Smith, D.W., Letourneau, E.J., Saunders, B.E., Kilpatrick, D.G., Resnick, H.S., and Best, C.L. (2000) "Delay in disclosure of childhood rape: Results from a national survey", *Child Abuse and Neglect* 24:273–287.

Smith, M., and Bentovim, A. (1994) "Sexual abuse", in M. Rutter and I. Hersov (Eds.) *Child and Adolescent Psychiatry: Modern Approaches* (3rd edition), Cambridge, MA: Blackwell Science.

Smucker, M.R., Dancu, C., Foa, E.B., and Niederee, J.L. (1995) "Imagery rescripting: A new treatment for survivors of childhood sexual abuse suffering from post-traumatic stress", *Journal of Cognitive Psychotherapy: An International Quarterly* 9:3–17.

Spacarelli, S., and Fuchs, C. (1997) "Variability in symptom expression among sexually abused girls: Developing multivariate models", *Journal of Clinical Child Psychology* 26:24–35.

Sroufe, L.A., Jacobvitz, D., Mangelsdorf, S., DeAngelo, E., and Ward, M.J. (1985) "Generational boundary dissolution between mothers and their preschool children: A relationships system approach", *Child Development* 56:317–325.

Stark, K. (1993) *Helping the Adult Survivor of Child Sexual Abuse: For Friends, Family, and Lovers*, Racine, WI: Mother Courage Press.

Stone, T.H., Winslade, W.J., and Klugman, C.M. (2000) "Sex offenders, sentencing laws and pharmaceutical treatment: A prescription for failure", *Behavioural Science and the Law* 18:83–110.

Taal, M., and Edelaar, M. (1997) "Positive and negative effects of a child sexual abuse prevention program", *Child Abuse and Neglect* 21:399–410.

Teasdale, J. (2000) "Prevention of relapse/recurrence in major depression by mindfulness-based cognitive therapy", *Journal of Consulting and Clinical Psychology* 68:615–623.

Ussher, J.M., and Dewberry, C. (1995) "The nature and long-term effects of childhood sexual abuse: A survey of adult women survivors in Britain", *British Journal of Clinical Psychology* 34:177–192.

Vogeltanz, N.D., Wilsnack, S.C., Harris, T.R., Wilsnack, R.W., Wonderlich, S.A., and Kristjanson, A.F. (1999) "Prevalence and risk factors for childhood sexual abuse in women: National survey findings", *Child Abuse and Neglect* 23:579–592.

Wagner, A.W., and Linehan, M.M. (1997) "Biosocial perspective on the relationship of childhood sexual abuse, suicidal behaviour, and borderline personality disorder", in M.C. Zanarini (Ed.) *Role of Sexual Abuse in the Aetiology of Borderline Personality Disorder*, Washington, DC: American Psychiatric Press.

Waldfogel, J. (2000) "Reforming child protective services", *Child Welfare* 79:43–57.

Walsh, B.W., and Rosen, P.M. (1985) "Self-mutilation and contagion: An empirical test", *American Journal of Psychiatry* 141:119–120.

Ward, A., Hudson, S.M., and Marshall, W.L. (1996) "Attachment style in sex offenders: A preliminary study", *Journal of Sex Research* 33:17–26.

Ward, A., Hudson, S.M., Marshall, W.L., and Siegert, R. (1995) "Attachment style and intimacy deficits in sexual offenders: A theoretical framework", *Sexual Abuse: A Journal of Research and Treatment* 7:317–335.

Warden, D. (1996) "The prevention of child sexual abuse", in W. Gilham and J. Thomson (Eds.) *Child Safety: Problem and Prevention from Preschool to Adolescence*, London: Routledge.

Weiss, E.L., Longhurst, J.G., and Mazure, C.M. (1999) "Childhood sexual abuse as a risk factor for depression in women: Psychological and neurological correlates", *American Journal of Psychiatry* 156:816–828.

Weissmann-Wind, T., and Silvern, L. (1994) "Parenting and family stress as mediators of the long-term effects of child abuse", *Child Abuse and Neglect* 18:439–453.

Welldon, E.V. (1988) *Mother, Madonna, Whore: The Idealisation and Denigration of Motherhood*, London: Free Association Books.

Wenninger, K., and Ehlers, A. (1998) "Dysfunctional cognitions and adult psychological functioning in child sexual abuse survivors", *Journal of Traumatic Stress* 11:281–300.

West, D. (1985) *Sexual Victimisations*, New York: Gower.

Westen, D., Ludolph, P., Misle, B., and Ruffins, S. (1990) "Physical and sexual abuse in adolescent girls with borderline personality disorder", *American Journal of Orthopsychiatry* 60:55–66.

Wilkins, P. (1999) "The relationship in person-centred counselling", in C. Feltham (Ed.) *Understanding the Counselling Relationship*, London: Sage.

Wilkins, R. (1990) "Women who sexually abuse children", *British Medical Journal* 300:1153–1154.

Williams, L.M. (1994) "Recall of childhood trauma: A retrospective study of women's memories of child sexual abuse", *Journal of Consulting and Clinical Psychology* 62:1167–1176.

Wills, F., and Sanders, D. (Eds.) (1997) *Cognitive Therapy: Transforming the Image*, London: Sage.

Winnicot, D. (1965) *The Maturational Process and the Facilitating Environment*, London: Hogarth.

Winnicot, D. (1986) *Home is Where we Start From: Essays by a Psychoanalyst*, Harmondsworth, Middlesex: Penguin.

Withers, J.M.J., and Mitchell, J. (1995) "False memory syndrome: Some reflections", *Clinical Psychology Forum*, 86:21–24.

Wolpe, J. (1958) *Psychotherapy by Reciprocal Inhibition*, Stanford: Stanford University Press.

Wolpe, J. (1969) *The Practice of Behaviour Therapy*, New York: Pergamon Press.

Wood, J.K. (1996) "The person-centred approach: Toward an understanding of its implication", in R. Hutterer, G. Pawlowsky, P.F. Schmid, and R. Stipsits (Eds.) *Client-Centred and Experiential Psychotherapy: A Paradigm in Motion*, Frankfurt-am-Main: Peter Lang.

Wurtele, S.K. (1999) "Comprehensiveness and collaboration: Key ingredients of an effective public health approach to preventing child sexual abuse", *Sexual Abuse: A Journal of Research and Treatment* 11:279–292.

Wyatt, G.E. (1985) "The sexual abuse of African American and European American women in childhood", *Child Abuse and Neglect* 9:507–519.

Wyatt, G.E., Burns-Loeb, T., Solis, B, and Vargas-Carmona, J. (1999) "The prevalence and circumstances of child sexual abuse: Changes across a decade", *Child Abuse and Neglect* 23:45–60.

Wyatt, G.E., and Peters, S.D. (1986a) "Issues in the definition of child sexual abuse in prevalence research", *Child Abuse and Neglect* 10:231–240.

Wyatt, G.E., and Peters, S.D. (1986b) "Methodological considerations in research on the prevalence of child abuse", *Child Abuse and Neglect* 10:241–251.

Yama, M.F., Tovey, S.L., and Fogas, B.S. (1993) "Childhood family environment and sexual abuse as predictors of anxiety and depression in adult women", *American Journal of Orthopsychiatry* 63:136–141.

Young, J.E. (1994) *Cognitive Therapy for Personality Disorders: A Schema Focused Approach*, Sarasota, Florida: Professional Resource Press.

Zanarini, M.C. (Ed.) (1997) *Role of Sexual Abuse in the Etiology of Borderline Personality Disorder*, Washington, DC: American Psychiatric Press.

Zanarini, M.C. (2000) "Childhood experiences associated with the development of borderline personality disorder", *The Psychiatric Clinics of North America* 23:89–101.

Zanarini, M.C., Dudo, E.D., Lewis, R.E., and Williams, A.A. (1997) "Childhood factors associated with the development of borderline personality disorder", in M.C. Zanarini (Ed.) *Role of Sexual Abuse in the Aetiology of Borderline Personality Disorder*, Washington, DC: American Psychiatric Press.

Zanarini, M.C., Gunderson, J.G., Frankenburg, F.R., and Chauncey, D.L. (1990) "Discriminating borderline personality disorder from other Axis II disorders", *American Journal of Psychiatry* 147:161–167.

Zanarini, M.C., Gunderson, J.G., Marino, M.F., Schwartz, E.O., and Frankenburg, F.R. (1989) "Childhood experiences of borderline patients", *Comprehensive Psychiatry* 30:18–25.

Zeanah, C.H. and Zeanah, P.D. (1989) "Intergenerational transmission of mal-treatment: Insights from attachment theory and research", *Psychiatry* 52:177–196.

Zweig-Frank, H., and Paris, J. (1997) "Relationship of sexual abuse to dissociation and self-mutilation in female patients", in M.C. Zanarini (Ed.) *Role of Sexual Abuse in the Etiology of Borderline Personality Disorder*, Washington, DC: American Psychiatric Press.

Index

Note: Page numbers in **bold** refer to figures and tables.